Sleep-Wrecked Kids

Helping parents raise happy, healthy kids, one sleep at a time

Sharon Moore

NEW YORK

LONDON • NASHVILLE • MELBOURNE • VANCOUVER

Sleep Wrecked Kids

Helping Parents Raise Happy, Healthy Kids, One Sleep at a Time

Published in New York, New York, by Morgan James Publishing. Morgan James is a trademark of Morgan James, LLC. www.MorganJamesPublishing.com

ISBN 9781642793963 paperback
ISBN 9781642793970 eBook
Library of Congress Control Number: 2018914371

Cover Design by:
Designerbility

Disclaimer

The material in this publication is of the nature of general comment only, and does not represent professional advice. It is not intended to provide specific guidance for particular circumstances and it should not be relied on as the basis for any decision to take action or not take action on any matter which it covers. Readers should obtain professional advice where appropriate, before making any such decision. To the maximum extent permitted by law, the author and publisher disclaim all responsibility and liability to any person, arising directly or indirectly from any person taking or not taking action based on the information in this publication.

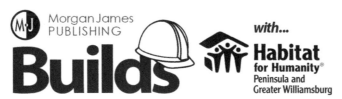

Morgan James is a proud partner of Habitat for Humanity Peninsula and Greater Williamsburg. Partners in building since 2006.

Get involved today! Visit
MorganJamesPublishing.com/giving-back

I dedicate this book to the men who have had a profound impact on my life:

My husband Andrew

My sons Max and Sam

My father, Patson John Brooks

who passed away on February 12, 2018 after a battle with melanoma

As a parent of three children, I've found conversations around sleep and children a minefield. There are so many different philosophies about what is best for my kids. Cutting through the confusion, *Sleep-Wrecked Kids* explains why good sleep is vital for kids' health and development – and what parents can do to help their kids achieve it.

A unique aspect of this book is its focus on the link between a child's upper airway and their sleep quality. Before reading *Sleep-Wrecked Kids*, I had given little thought to airway health and the role it could be playing in my kids' sleep troubles – or my own. Many children's sleep books focus on behaviours and routines alone, but these are just part of the picture. This book is packed full of advice to help parents identify breathing issues, exercises for developing better airway health and guidance on where to seek professional help for disordered sleep.

Sharon Moore has an outstanding passion for helping parents and kids get the sleep they need. My family has made some changes since reading *Sleep-Wrecked Kids*, and we're looking forward to reaping the benefits of better sleep!

Jenny Riddle
Mild snorer and parent of three snuffly sleepers

In *Sleep-Wrecked Kids,* Sharon Moore explains the sleep needs of children and the consequences of poor sleep and shows readers how to make a plan that will get children the sleep they need to live a better quality life.

Sharon first takes a behavioural approach to optimising children's routines and environments to improve their sleep. She then explains the role that orofacial myofunctional therapy can play in creating a healthy airway. This is a vital topic to cover. The available evidence-based data shows that orofacial myofunctional therapy plays a very important role in keeping the airway open in the treatment of obstructive sleep apnoea. It is a non-invasive, educational approach to treatment.

This book addresses all the aspects related to the importance of sleep for the healthy development of children in a clear and detailed manner, showing the author's vast expertise in this field. Surely, this book is a jewel in the field of health care for a better sleep.

Esther Mandelbaum Gonçalves Bianchini, SLP, PhD
Professor, Post Graduation Program of Pontifical Catholic University of São Paulo
Coordinator, SLP Commission of the Brazilian Sleep Society

As a speech language pathologist myself, treating patients with sleep disorders related to other symptoms, I found *Sleep-Wrecked Kids* easy to read and useful, with its charts, questionnaires, quotes and statistics. Kids with allergies and upper airway problems are often misdiagnosed as having behavioural or educational issues when, in fact, the likely cause is the impact of allergies and anatomical, physiological and psychological factors on nocturnal breathing.

Kudos to Sharon for writing a much-needed book for parents and professionals alike. It should be available in every health professional's waiting room and to every group where parents gather together to share and support each other.

Licia Coceani Paskay, MS, CCC-SLP
Speech language pathologist, Los Angeles, California

This book will help guide the future generation to become genetically as healthy as possible. The importance of sleep for a child's proper growth and development and all aspects of health should not be taken lightly. *Sleep-Wrecked Kids* will help to inform parents how to enable the growth of a proper airway, thereby facilitating proper dental development. This will enhance many issues that modern society is using medication, surgery, repeated orthodontics, and treating the symptoms instead of the cause.

Periodontal diseases, jaw (TMJ) pain, sleep disorders and cavities are some problems that dentists address today. Many of these issues are best treated with therapy that enables proper breathing, chewing and swallowing and the elimination of oral habits that interfere with the body's normal function and development. As a dental hygienist, my job is to *prevent* dental diseases. I feel the answers to so many problems are found in this book.

Joy Moeller, RDH, BS | USA
Dental hygienist and orofacial myofunctional therapist
Founder and instructor teaching myofunctional therapy for the AOMT

Sleep and breathing seem simple, but supporting children and families with sleep disorders and breathing disorders can feel very complex. Sharon Moore shares the current data in a parent-friendly way, explaining dysfunction, the impact on development, the consequences of inaction and how to find help. I can't wait to share it with my patients and their families.

Linda D'Onofrio, MS, CCC-SLP

Sleep-Wrecked Kids is truly needed for parents and professionals. There are more babies and children with sleep problems than ever before. These disorders are usually related to difficulties in airway development and breathing patterns. Some problems may even begin in utero.

Beyond this, we see structural and functional disorders likely related to current child-rearing practices: For example, many babies spend an inordinate amount of their awake time on their backs, impeding their development of foundational postural control and proper jaw growth. Additionally, bottles, spouted cups, and pacifiers appear to impede mouth and airway development. On top of it all, we are likely seeing epigenetic changes in our species due to these practices.

Sharon Moore addresses these important issues, among others, in her book. I want to thank Sharon for taking the time to explain the causes and resolutions for airway and sleep disorders in children.

Diane Bahr, MS, CCC-SLP, CIMI
International presenter on feeding, motor-speech and mouth development
Author of *Nobody Ever Told Me (or My Mother) That!: Everything from Bottles and Breathing to Healthy Speech Development*

When a baby is born, and even before, one of the parents' major concerns is: 'Is my baby going to sleep well?' Nowadays, clinicians and the research community know that sleep disorders have a negative influence on children's craniofacial and behavioural development.

Parents have a crucial role identifying the first signs that something isn't right. *Sleep-Wrecked Kids* helps parents recognise these signs and shows clearly what can be done. It is an important guide to promoting better airway, dental and behavioural development for all children. The orofacial myofunctional strategies and intervention programs are a simple but, as recent research shows, effective adjunctive treatment for sleep-breathing disorders. It has clear but rigorous language that allows all the readers to understand sleep and breathing behaviour better and implement actions that can promote better health.

As a father, speech and language therapist (SLP) and researcher, I can only say one thing: congratulations Sharon Moore! This book is an excellent resource for parents and clinicians of different fields. SLP, medical and dental professionals will all benefit from reading it.

Ricardo Santos, SLT, MSc, PhD
Speech and language therapist
Co-Founder of the Portuguese Society of TMJ and Orofacial Pain

As a father of young adults, I wish this book was available when my sons were little. If I could have read only one book to help me be a better parent, it would have to be this one. I knew sleep was everything, but I did not know the real impact, both short and long term, of sleep issues. Nor could I identify them.

In hindsight I now see so much unnecessary angst was experienced through my lack of understanding about sleep. I feel I would have provided much better support and nurturing for the entire family with the knowledge and practical advice this book provides.

I am astounded at the depth of academic rigour and research included in "Sleep Wrecked Kids", yet it reads so easily and clearly for a parent like me. It is simply compelling, and I am surprised there is not more focus placed on what is clearly a near-epidemic of sleep issues amongst our children – and ourselves.

Do yourself and your loved ones a favour. Read this book more than once, heed the advice, and act. I wish I did.

Charles Babylone, Regretful Dad

Contents

Foreword

Sleep-disordered breathing in a child is often worrying, and the associated behavioural and school problems are stressful for the whole family. With recognition of the importance of obstructive sleep apnoea (OSA) in children, practice guidelines have been developed for the management of OSA in the USA and Europe. A panel of experts in paediatric OSA in Asia recently prepared a position statement for management of childhood OSA in Asia. The purpose of this statement is to provide a reference standard in the diagnosis and management of childhood OSA for doctors working in Asia. This shows how important this health issue has become.

There is a need for greater awareness of sleep disorders, particularly sleep-disordered breathing, among parents and the wider community. This is so that the urgency and gravity of sleep as a treatable public health issue is better understood and addressed effectively.

Sharon contributes greatly to this aim with her book, *Sleep-Wrecked Kids*. Sharon is a speech pathologist with years of experience in treating OSA in children. In this book, Sharon provides practical suggestions and facts for handling 'sleep-wrecked kids'. This book addresses the importance of sleep and the impact of a child's airway on the quality of their sleep. Sharon also highlights measures that can prevent the development of OSA and talks about the benefits of orofacial myofunctional therapy – an unknown among most health care workers and the lay public. She also stresses the importance of nasal breathing, which is an important step in the prevention of OSA.

This is an easy-to-read book that empowers the parents to identify the sleep issues and the simple steps that make a huge difference for any sleep-wrecked kid and their sleep-wrecked family.

Daniel Ng, MBBS, MD
Founding President, Asian Paediatric Pulmonology Society
Certified Sleep Disorders Specialist, World Association of Sleep Medicine

A note for our North American readers

Please keep in mind that this book has been written in Australian English, so some of the spellings and terms might seem a bit unusual.

Two of these are 'dummies', which is our term for pacifiers, and 'nappies', which is our term for diapers. All Latin terms use the Australian spelling, such as sleep anpoea (rather than sleep apnea), and other spelling anomalies include words like colour, organise, realise and so on.

Introduction

Sally's sleep is in trouble.

Sally breathes through her mouth constantly as she sleeps, tossing and turning all night long. She seems to have periods where she stops breathing and then snorts herself awake. Although Sally sleeps in her own bed, she often wakes in fear, so either mum or dad will sleep in her bed with her. They need to take this in turns because she rolls, snores and kicks so much that they hardly get any sleep when lying next to her. Sally is such a restless sleeper that when her mum is working late in her home office, which shares a wall with her daughter's bedroom, she can hear Sally bang into the wall around three times an hour as she tosses and turns. There is constant drool on her pillowcase, which they change a couple of times a week.

While her twin sister has been successfully night-time toilet trained, Sally will wet her bed every second night or so and doesn't wake up for hours after the wetting. She is so sad when this happens that her parents have reverted to giving her night-time nappies. Unfortunately, this also causes her distress, despite their reassurances that she is loved and still their big girl.

During the day, Sally continues to breathe mainly through her mouth. She speaks so nasally that most people cannot understand what she says. She was slow to speak compared to her twin, who still does a lot of the talking for her. Her parents have tried nasal cleaning and nasal sprays but to no avail.

Sally is a loving and beautiful kid who just wants to please everyone, yet this sleeping and breathing problem seems to affect her ability to concentrate. She is constantly tired.

Sally has the hallmarks of sleep apnoea.

But Sally isn't the only child struggling with challenging and worrying sleep problems. When Adam Mansbach's book *Go the F**k to Sleep* debuted at number one on the *New York Times* bestseller list, it surprised everyone.[1] Yet Mansbach's raw, honest and hilarious verses capture so aptly the sentiments of every parent who has experienced the frustration of overtired, under-slept children, whose stalling tactics at bedtime have stretched parents' patience to the limit. In fact, it hit such a chord that it has sold over 1.5 million copies worldwide as I write.

The response to Mansbach's irreverent book has helped to reveal the widespread nature of poor sleep among children and parents. And it's verified by the data. Up to twenty-four per cent of all children, and thirty-five per cent of children under two years of age, have frequent problems sleeping.[2] These are, most commonly, behavioural sleep problems; psychologist Sarah Blunden estimates that thirty to forty per cent of children's sleep problems are related to habits and behaviours.[3] However, many more of these sleep issues are physiological and will have long-term consequences. Leading paediatric sleep specialist Judith Owens and psychologist Jodi Mindell report that twenty-five per cent of all children experience some type of sleep problem at some point during childhood.[4]

As a rule, the more serious the disorder is, the more severe the symptoms. At one end of the spectrum, parents may wonder why their kids are so tired and grumpy. They may wonder why they can't concentrate, and why they're acting out, possibly aggressive. They may wonder why they're doing poorly in school. It's especially deceiving with super smart kids, because they seem to be doing well, but they are simply not doing anywhere near their best. Parents may be so used to their child being this way, they never imagine it could be any different.

1   Adam Mansbach and Ricardo Cortés, *Go the F**k to Sleep*, (New York, NY: Akashic Books, 2011).

2   Olivero Bruni, 'Insomnia: Clinical and Diagnostic Aspects', *World Sleep Society Conference* (Prague, 2017).

3   Sarah Blunden, 'Behavioural Sleep Disorders across the Developmental Age Span: An Overview of Causes, Consequences and Treatment Modalities', *Psychology*, no. 3 (2012): 249–56, https://doi.org/10.4236/psych.2012.33035.

4   Judith Owens and Jodi Mindell, *Take Charge of Your Child's Sleep: The All-In-One Resource for Solving Sleep Problems in Kids and Teens* (New York: Marlowe & Co., 2005).

At the other end of the spectrum lie the diagnosable sleep disorders. And there are over ninety of them. One such class of sleep disorders is sleep-disordered breathing (SDB), which can affect kids' brains, hearts, blood pressure, growth, appetites, teeth and jaw development.[5] Then there's obstructive sleep apnoea (OSA), the severe end of sleep-disordered breathing. Kids with OSA struggle to function and stay awake, causing significant behaviour and learning problems, speech delays and mood problems. Kids with OSA have difficulty following directions and are five times more likely to be diagnosed with ADHD. What's more, ninety-five per cent of children with OSA are never diagnosed.[6]

>> ninety-five per cent of children with OSA are never diagnosed

Regardless of the cause of a sleep problem and whether it is mild, moderate or severe, poor sleep will impact on how kids are able to function in many areas of life, because disrupted sleep means a disruption of the vital restorative brain processes that are supposed to happen during sleep.

And when kids can't sleep, neither can their parents – leaving them short on patience, unable to perform well at work and unable to be the parents they want to be.

Why isn't anyone doing anything?

Many parents, though they might notice symptoms like snoring, noisy breathing and night waking, assume that these are normal. This is a problem. The truth is that these symptoms are *not* normal. Common, yes, but not normal.

Take snoring, for instance. According to Dr Jim Papadopoulos, a paediatric sleep specialist, snoring is 'like having a plug in your throat that's

---

5   David McIntosh, *Snored to Death: Are You Dying in Your Sleep?* (Maroochydore: ENT Specialists Australia, 2017).

6   Leila Kheirandish-Gozal, 'Morbidity of OSA in Children', *World Sleep Society Conference* (Prague, 2017).

stopping air (and therefore oxygen) getting to the brain. It has effects on behaviour, learning and mood. Kids (even when they are mild mannered and doing well at day care or school) will have trouble concentrating. Studies show a drop of ten points on IQ tests'.[7] Those little snuffles and snorts might sound cute, but they could be doing real, long-term damage.

Even if parents do realise that their kid has a problem, many just want to find a quick fix. All of us are busy and tired, and having a sleep-wrecked kid makes it worse. It's no wonder we want to find the path of least resistance, like fixing snoring with a pillow under the head or playing musical beds in the middle of the night to help settle a child.

>> the right kind of help is not always easy to find

Some parents do take the next step and look for expert help. However, the right kind of help is not always easy to find. The options are confusing and the advice given conflicting. Diagnosing a sleep disorder is a very specialised area of medicine – to the point that many doctors and health professionals don't know how to recognise or fix it. One of my clients visited *twenty-three* medical specialists in Australia and the US before finding the right type of help for her child. Some other parents I know took their child to the doctor, reporting that their child was always tired. The doctor's advice? 'Get more exercise or try to relax more.' The sleep was never addressed. Some professionals even argue that sleep doesn't matter and that children can be trained to need less. Different health professionals vary widely in their advice and approach, leaving parents unsure about who to listen to and what to do.

Unsurprisingly, many parents give up. Sleep goes into the 'too hard' basket. Some families discover that they can't find a solution because parents themselves are unable to agree on the way to handle it. Others settle into a kind of resigned complacency: 'We tried everything and it didn't work, so I guess that's just the way it is.'

7   Jim Papadopoulos, 'Another Sleepless Night', Yahoo7, interview transcript, last edited July 22, 2013, https://au.news.yahoo.com/sunday-night/a/18093130/another-sleepless-night.

It doesn't have to be this way...

Sleep problems are serious, with the consequences reaching far beyond the daily frustration they cause for the family. When kids don't get the rest they need night after night, the four key domains for development, physical (growth, immunity), mental (IQ, focus, problem solving), emotional (mood and emotional regulation) and social, are all affected. Simply, sleep-wrecked kids can never be at their best, and neither can their parents.

>> I want to encourage you to become the lifeguard of your kids' sleep

What can you do?

In this book, I want to encourage you to become the lifeguard of your kids' sleep. Lifeguards watch for danger, protect swimmers and prevent drowning. Parents do the same thing – guiding, protecting, nourishing and caring for their children in all areas of their lives. They also rescue when required.

As a parent, you are the right person to be a lifeguard in your kids' lives. From birth until now, you've seen them every day and have always been the first one to notice any little change. This means you are perfectly positioned to identify the signs and symptoms of sleep problems.

However, in order to be that lifeguard, you need good information and support from the time your kids are born. If your children are older, though, don't panic – it's never too late to start!

In this book, I'm going to take you behind the scenes of your children's sleep so you can understand why sleep is so important, what to look out for and what practical tools you can use to help your kids get a good night's rest. In the coming chapters, you'll discover:

THE IMPORTANCE OF SLEEP

We'll start by sharing why good sleep is so important and how bad sleep affects your kids' behaviour, physical health and mental aptitude. We'll also touch on the long-term, cumulative effects of sleep deprivation, as well as covering the issue of sleep deprivation for kids with special needs.

UNDERSTANDING DISORDERED SLEEP

To be the best lifeguard you can be, you need to become 'sleep literate', developing an understanding of what constitutes good sleep and bad sleep. We will debunk some common sleep myths along the way. This chapter will also share how good sleep works, the ways in which sleep disorders disrupt it, and the most common causes of disordered sleep.

RECOGNISING THE RED FLAGS

To be a great lifeguard, you'll need to recognise the key signs that your kid is not hitting the right sleep formula. These signs are usually staring you in the face; in fact, some of them are literally 'in your face'.[8] In this chapter, you'll learn how to identify the red flags that indicate your children are not getting the sleep they need and determine whether further action is necessary.

WHAT YOU CAN DO TO HELP YOUR KIDS SLEEP

If your kids are struggling with disordered sleep, there's good news. Much can be done, starting with changes you can make to your child's physical environment, emotional environment and routines throughout the day and night.

HOW TO BUILD A HEALTHY AIRWAY, THE 'MYO' WAY

When changes to your kids' routine and environment don't solve the problem, it's time to look deeper. The second most common sleep disorder is related to the upper airway and how well the muscles keep the airway open. Myofunctional therapy is the systematic training of the muscles of the upper airway.

---

8 Sharon Moore, 'Sleep Disorders Are in Your Face', in *The 2nd AAMS Congress* (Chicago, 2017).

In this chapter, you'll discover the essential early life activities that will ensure these muscles develop properly, and how myofunctional therapy will be able to help if things aren't working as they should (at any age).

WHEN TO BRING IN A SPECIALIST

If your child has a sleep disorder, or changes to their environment and routine aren't working, it's time to bring in the experts. Signs and symptoms of serious sleep disorder should be addressed by medical specialists. In this chapter, I'll outline who can help, how they can help, and how to find the right team members to help your kids get the sleep they need.

Who am I?

As a parent, I know how distressing it is when children are out of sorts and you feel helpless to fix it. There's nothing like lack of sleep to bring out the worst in kids and their parents. I also know that when good sleep is the norm, kids and their families can grow and thrive.

I'm the founder of Well Spoken, a speech pathology and orofacial myofunctional practice in Canberra, Australia. I've been working as a speech pathologist for over thirty-eight years and have conducted over 40,000 clinical consultations. I've seen first-hand how sleep problems interfere with kids' health and family happiness. That's why I want to help parents recognise and fix kids' sleep problems.

> **» 700,000 Aussie kids under 10 have sleep problems, which goes up to 1.9 million in the UK, 11 million in the USA and 1/4 of a billion in Asia**

As research in sleep medicine proliferates, so does our understanding of poor sleep and its many consequences. If we just look at kids under age ten, there are 1.9 million in the UK, eleven million in the USA, one quarter of a billion kids across Asia, and 700,000 Aussie kids who have sleep problems, and these are conservative figures based on twenty-five per cent of the population. Sadly, many are misdiagnosed or missed altogether.

Kids with sleep problems can be sleep deprived and even oxygen deprived. It's much more than just feeling foggy the next day. As a speech pathologist, I quickly discovered how sleep affects communication, learning, focus and behaviour. Sleep-wrecked kids are poorly behaved, unhappy and not alert, and are easily misdiagnosed with ADHD. These kids start school behind their peers and it's really hard for them to catch up, causing ripple effects that last a lifetime. I began to wonder how any therapy for language or learning problems could be effective unless kids (and parents) were properly rested.

Sleep specialists around the globe are calling for parents to have a greater understanding of sleep problems. That's why I wrote *Sleep-Wrecked Kids*: to help parents better understand the consequences of poor sleep and to give them strategies, not only to recognise when their own kids are 'sleep-wrecked', but to actually turn that sleep around.

>> Every parent should have this health topic firmly on their radar, so every kid has the best chance of getting the sleep they need and deserve every night

My mission is to spread the word among parents so that every parent has this health topic firmly on their radar, and every kid has the best chance of getting the sleep they need and deserve every night. By doing this, our collective efforts may even raise global IQ, happiness and health.

I believe that parents deserve to have the latest knowledge at their fingertips for treatable health issues. Kids deserve to grow well, be happy and be the very best version of themselves. Every time I talk with parents, that's exactly what they want for their kids too. Let's face it; everyone deserves a good night's sleep. *Sleep-Wrecked Kids* will help this happen – for you *and* your kids.

CHAPTER ONE

The importance of sleep

Sleep problems have tripled in the last ten years.
It's a big social problem and affects the whole family.

DR O. BRUNI[9]

>> This is a book about sleep-wrecked kids. But I want to begin the conversation by talking about sleep-wrecked adults

This is a book about sleep-wrecked kids. But I want to begin the conversation by talking about sleep-wrecked adults.

Adults have their own challenges with sleep, and on top of that, when kids don't sleep well, neither do the parents. According to a survey conducted by the Centre for Disease Control and Prevention, more than thirty-five per cent of Americans sleep less than seven hours in a typical day.[10] Meanwhile, thirty per cent of adults average less than six hours of sleep per day.[11]

Our modern culture often focuses on productivity over rest. Slogans like 'sleep is for wimps' and 'I'll sleep when I'm dead' are commonplace. The truth is, however, that more waking hours can cause you to become *less* productive. Sleep debt is not a mere inconvenience; additional wakefulness has a neurobiological cost, which accumulates over time.[12]

9   Bruni, 'Insomnia: Clinical and Diagnostic Aspects'.
10   Institute of Medicine, 'Sleep Disorders and Sleep Deprivation: An Unmet Public Health Problem', (Washington, DC: National Academic Press, 2006), https://doi.org/10.17226/11617.
11   C.A. Schoenborn and P.F. Adams, 'Health Behaviors of Adults: United States, 2005–2007', *Vital Health Stat* 10, no. 245 (March 2010).
12   Hans P.A. van Dongen, Greg Maislin, Janet M. Mullington and David F. Dinges, 'The Cumulative Cost of Additional Wakefulness: Dose-Response Effects on Neurobehavioral Functions and Sleep Physiology from Chronic Sleep Restriction and Total Sleep Deprivation', *Sleep* 26, no. 2 (1 March 2003): 117–26, https://doi.org/10.1093/sleep/26.2.117.

When sleep deprived, your body struggles to extract glucose from the blood stream and your brain is unable to think straight. This then impacts your rational thinking, willpower, self-control, productivity and interactions with colleagues – so this can be very bad in the work place. In fact, sleeping fewer than six hours a night or more than eight leads to low scores on logical thinking and vocabulary, along with ageing your brain.[13]

Even small amounts of sleep deprivation degrade your abilities and put you into a state where you may fall into micro sleeps – a state to which you are oblivious. This is a dangerous state to be in while driving a car, wielding a scalpel or operating machinery, and it can happen at any time of the day. A lack of sleep has been linked to motor vehicle crashes, industrial disasters, and medical and other occupational errors.[14,15] Even the Chernobyl meltdown and the Challenger space shuttle disaster have been linked to sleep deprivation.[16,17]

Dangerously, most sleep-impaired individuals believe their ability to perform these tasks is at its usual standard, when tests show it is not. One study showed that subjects sleeping six hours or fewer per night were as impaired in their daytime cognitive performance as if they'd completely missed two nights of sleep. Yet these adults were not aware that they were impaired at all and thought they were fine: 'Sleepiness ratings suggest that subjects were largely unaware of these increasing cognitive deficits, which may explain why the impact of chronic sleep restriction on waking cognitive functions is often assumed to be benign.'[18]

13   Richard Wiseman, *Night School: The Life-Changing Science of Sleep* (London: Pan Books, 2015).

14   Institute of Medicine, 'Sleep Disorders and Sleep Deprivation: An Unmet Public Health Problem'.

15   National Highway Traffic Safety Administration, Drowsy Driving and Automobile Crashes: Report and Recommendations, (Washington, DC: U.S. Department of Transportation, 1998), https://www.nhtsa.gov/sites/nhtsa.dot.gov/files/808707.pdf.

16   Merrill M. Mitler, Mary A. Carskadon, Charles A. Czeisier, William C. Dement, David F. Dinges and R. Curtis Graeber, 'Catastrophes, Sleep, and Public Policy: Consensus Report', *Sleep* 11, no. 1 (1988): 100–09, https://doi.org/10.1093/sleep/11.1.100.

17   James K. Walsh, William C. Dement, and David F. Dinges, 'Sleep Medicine, Public Policy, and Public Health', *Principles and Practice of Sleep Medicine*, no. 4 (2005): 648–56, https://doi.org/10.1016/b0-72-160797-7/50060-4.

18   Dongen, Maislin, Mullington and Dinges, 'The Cumulative Cost of Additional Wakefulness', 117–26.

>> When people are sleepy, they perceive their performance is normal when in fact it is not. Not even close

When people are sleepy, they perceive their performance is normal when in fact it is not. Not even close.

Beyond issues of performance and productivity, sleep deprivation has profound effects on many areas of physical and mental health. Surrey University scientists discovered that over 700 of the body's genes, or the expression of those genes, are altered when someone regularly gets less than six hours of sleep a night over one week.[19]

Research around sleep fragmentation and disturbed sleep demonstrates links to cancer.[20,21] Further, the risk of pancreatic, lung, kidney and skin cancers is significantly higher in patients with obstructive sleep apnoea.[22]

There are even studies now linking diabetes, schizophrenia, heart attacks, stroke and Alzheimer's with sleep deprivation and fragmented sleep. In fact, sleeping five or fewer hours per night instead of the recommended seven to nine hours for adults may increase mortality risk by as much as fifteen per cent.[23]

Extreme experiments in sleep deprivation were conducted during the 1950s. In one case, a young man who stayed awake for eight days demonstrated increasingly erratic behaviour. As the subject tried to stay awake,

19   C. S. Moller-Levet, S. N. Archer, G. Bucca, E. E. Laing, A. Slak, R. Kabiljo, J. C. Y. Lo, N. Santhi, M. Von Schantz, C. P. Smith, and D.-J. Dijk, 'Effects of Insufficient Sleep on Circadian Rhythmicity and Expression Amplitude of the Human Blood Transcriptome', *Proceedings of the National Academy of Sciences* 110, no. 12 (2013), https://doi.org/10.1073/pnas.1217154110.

20   F. Javier Nieto, Paul E. Peppard, Terry Young, Laurel Finn, Khin Mae Hla, and Ramon Farré, 'Sleep-Disordered Breathing and Cancer Mortality', *American Journal of Respiratory and Critical Care Medicine* 186, no. 2 (2012): 190–94, https://doi.org/10.1164/rccm.201201-0130oc.

21   Francisco Campos-Rodriguez, Miguel A. Martinez-Garcia, Montserrat Martinez, Joaquin Duran-Cantolla, Monica De La Peña, María J. Masdeu, Monica Gonzalez, Felix Del Campo, Inmaculada Gallego, Jose M. Marin, Ferran Barbe, Jose M. Montserrat and Ramon Farre, 'Association between Obstructive Sleep Apnea and Cancer Incidence in a Large Multicenter Spanish Cohort', *American Journal of Respiratory and Critical Care Medicine* 187, no. 1 (2013): 99–105, https://doi.org/10.1164/rccm.201209-1671oc.

22   David Gozal, 'Sleep Apnea and Cancer: Illicit Partnerships', in *AACP Australian Chapter – 6th International Symposium*, (Sydney, March 18, 2017).

23   Institute of Medicine, 'Sleep Disorders and Sleep Deprivation: An Unmet Public Health Problem'.

he developed delusions, like his shoes being full of spiders, and paranoia, thinking a visiting doctor was an undertaker.[24] Throughout the experiment, which would be impermissible today, he also suffered psychotic episodes, moodiness, depression, lethargy, slurred speech and aggression. Such extreme sleep deprivation, which is associated with ongoing insomnia, has been shown to trigger long-term psychological instability like paranoia, confusion, delusion, hallucination, moodiness and memory issues.[25]

So if you are wondering why you are cranky, suspicious and reacting like a cat on a hot tin roof, it may just be related to sleep deprivation.

>> very few people see that they may be torturing *themselves* by not getting the right amount of sleep each night

Although it's well known that sleep deprivation is a torture technique that can lead to hallucination and coercive lying, very few people see that they may be torturing *themselves* by not getting the right amount of sleep each night, whether by under- or overdoing it. 'Short sleepers' are people who report sleeping fewer than seven hours on average per night and 'long sleepers' are individuals sleep more than nine hours on a typical night.[26] Research indicates that both are at increased risk of all-cause mortality.[27] Interestingly, 'excessive daytime napping might be a useful marker of increased respiratory risk'.[28]

Night-time urination, otherwise known as nocturia, is a bi-product of night-time airway obstruction and appears to be a risk factor for earlier

24   Wiseman, *Night School: The Life-Changing Science of Sleep.*
25   John J. Ross, 'Neurological Findings after Prolonged Sleep Deprivation', *Archives of Neurology* 12, no. 4 (1965): 399–403, https://doi.org/10.1001/archneur.1965.00460280069006.
26   Lisa Gallicchio and Bindu Kalesan, 'Sleep Duration and Mortality: A Systematic Review and Meta-Analysis', *Journal of Sleep Research* 18, no. 2 (2009): 148–58, https://doi.org/10.1111/j.1365-2869.2008.00732.x.
27   Ibid.
28   Yue Leng, Nick W. J. Wainwright, Francesco P. Cappuccio, Paul G. Surtees, Shabina Hayat, Robert Luben, Carol Brayne and Kay-Tee Khaw, 'Daytime Napping and Increased Risk of Incident Respiratory Diseases: Symptom, Marker, or Risk Factor?' *Sleep Medicine* 23 (2016): 12–15, https://doi.org/10.1016/j.sleep.2016.06.012.

death. Airway obstruction means the heart has to work harder to breathe, releasing a hormone called atrial natriuretic factor, which impacts kidney function and leads to night-time urination. In fact, men between twenty and forty-nine years of age who wake to urinate more than twice a night have double the risk of dying than other men their age.[29] Night-time urination acts as a red flag, signalling health and possible airway issues, and may be marker for increased risk of coronary heart disease.[30] Thankfully, dealing with sleep and breathing problems can see a reduction or elimination of this problem.[31] During normal calm breathing and sleep, urination is inhibited by a hormone called antidiuretic hormone. Of course, there may be other influencing factors, like too many fluids before bed or a tiny bladder, but if these are not your problem, airway and disturbed breathing is a likely culprit.

>> beauty sleep is a real thing

Even when we take a step back from the grave health risks, poor sleep affects quality of life at a fundamental level. Your face reflects your sleep. The stress hormone cortisol is released with sleep deprivation; several nights of poor sleep can prevent the production of collagen and increase fine lines and dark circles around the eyes. Chronic sleep deprivation increases the signs of ageing and lowers your satisfaction in your appearance.[32,33] It turns out that beauty sleep is a real thing. Sleep problems are literally 'in your face'.

29 Steven Park, '7 Surprising Health Conditions That Can Be from Poor Breathing at Night', December 6, 2017, podcast, MP3 audio, http://doctorstevenpark.com/7conditions#more-11214.

30 Deborah J. Lightner, Amy E. Krambeck, Debra J. Jacobson, Michaela E. Mcgree, Steven J. Jacobsen, Michael M. Lieber, Véronique L. Roger, Cynthia J. Girman and Jennifer L. St. Sauver, 'Nocturia is Associated with an Increased Risk of Coronary Heart Disease and Death', BJU International 110, no. 6 (2012): 848–53, https://doi.org/10.1111/j.1464-410x.2011.10806.x.

31 M. G. Umlauf and E. R. Chasens, 'Sleep Disordered Breathing and Nocturnal Polyuria: Nocturia and Enuresis', Sleep Med Rev 7, no. 5 (2003): 403–11.

32 P. Oyetakin-White, A. Suggs, B. Koo, M. S. Matsui, D. Yarosh, K. D. Cooper, and E. D. Baron, 'Does Poor Sleep Quality Affect Skin Ageing?' Clinical and Experimental Dermatology 40, no. 1 (2014): 17–22, https:/doi.org/10.1111/ced.12455.

33 J. Axelsson, T. Sundelin, M. Ingre, E. J. W. Van Someren, A. Olsson, and M. Lekander, 'Beauty Sleep: Experimental Study on the Perceived Health and Attractiveness of Sleep Deprived People', British Medical Journal 341, no. 14/2 (2010): C6614, https://doi.org/10.1136/bmj.c6614.

>> When sleep deprived, you feel hungrier than you actually are, do not feel full when you should, and are more likely to reach for carbohydrate-dense food. This is a triple whammy for weight gain!

Sleep deprivation even has an impact on shopping habits, with sleep-deprived people buying more junk food than those who are properly rested. The hormones leptin and ghrelin send signals to the brain about hunger and satiety. Leptin tells you when you are full, and ghrelin tells you when you are hungry. Both leptin and ghrelin are disrupted by poor sleep. This means that you feel hungrier than you actually are and you do not feel full when you should. Adding to that, we are more likely to reach for carbohydrate-dense food when tired.[34] This is a triple whammy for weight gain!

If chronic sleep deprivation is bad for us individually, it's also bad for us collectively. Economically, the price of untreated sleep disorders is very high to society. In the US, the twenty-three million adults with moderate to severe obstructive sleep apnoea (OSA) cost the government between $65 billion and $165 billion *annually*.[35] The costs related to leaving OSA untreated are diverse and include health treatments, poor work performance, work absence, depression, relationship breakdown, motor vehicle accidents and occupational errors.

The less you sleep, the more you are awake. The severity of chronic sleep restriction and total sleep deprivation has a direct bearing on how well you behave, make decisions and solve problems in daily life. And this is just how sleep deprivation affects adults!

Unfortunately, the effects of sleep deprivation can be even more disastrous for kids.

---

34 Sebastian M. Schmid, Manfred Hallschmid, Kamila Jauch-Chara, Jan Born and Bernd Schultes, 'A Single Night of Sleep Deprivation Increases Ghrelin Levels and Feelings of Hunger in Normal-Weight Healthy Men', *Journal of Sleep Research* 17, no. 3 (2008): 331–34, https://doi.org/10.1111/j.1365-2869.2008.00662.x.

35 'The Price of Fatigue', Harvard Medical School, PDF document, December 2010, https://sleep.med.harvard.edu/file_download/100.

How sleep problems are hurting your kids

When kids don't, won't or can't go to sleep, wake frequently in the night or have difficulty going back to sleep, there are daytime consequences that can look different to the adult ones – behaviourally, physically and mentally. The effects can be subtle or very obvious, and these compound over time. Some kids become tired but wired, while others become lethargic and poorly coordinated. Some may appear to be okay but are, in fact, operating way below their ability level.

Behavioural consequences of sleep problems

Four-year-old Daniel had turned into a little monster. Daniel had been a poor sleeper from birth. He refused to go to bed at night, woke his parents frequently and only had seven hours of sleep a night (instead of the recommended ten to thirteen hours for his age). He never slept for more than two hours at a stretch. During the day, he wouldn't take naps.

Like many sleep-deprived kids, every day Daniel would hit the ground running, reacting to sleep deprivation with over-activity, which the body craves as compensation for poor sleep. Not only that, but Daniel had an explosive temper and was extremely defiant.

After two years of Daniel's irrational meltdowns, his poor parents were at breaking point (and so was their marriage). His mum told me, 'I can't be the nice mummy I want to be or the one he deserves. I'm too tired.'

She saw more than twenty-three medical specialists in Australia and the US, and it wasn't until a dentist recognised an airway issue that they made some progress.

When I saw Daniel, he had the hallmarks of a sleep breathing disorder: problems with his breathing muscles, underdeveloped upper and lower jaws, dark circles under his eyes, lip tie and a tongue-tie.[36] He also had a long, narrow facial structure, which is frequently associated with a smaller airway.

Looking at how his face, mouth and throat muscles were working, I could see some problems. Daniel usually had his tongue out and forward while mouth breathing, had a habit of licking his lips and didn't chew his food properly. This was a strong indication that the upper airway muscles were not working as they should to support an open airway. He was also very fussy with food, to the extent that he would only eat nine foods. And he was small for his age, suffered from seasonal allergies, had a habitual cough, would grind his teeth and was very, very anxious. To top it off, his speech was delayed.

All in all, Daniel was one tired little puppy.

Despite visits to so many medical specialists, no one had seriously considered that Daniel's tonsils and adenoids might be part of the problem. As it turned out, both tonsils and adenoids were enlarged and leading to airway obstruction and snoring. This could explain why he woke frequently and was unable to go into deeper sleep cycles.[37] Given this, it was also plausible that the tonsils and adenoids contributed to blockages in the airway at night, creating negative pressure in the airway, pulling up acid from his stomach and causing reflux symptoms. While it appeared he did not have the more serious signs of OSA (gasping, choking and breathing stoppages), he was snoring and his sleep was disrupted by multiple wakings and arousals, which meant there was no way he could achieve the deep, restful sleep he needed to grow and thrive.

When Daniel's tonsils and adenoids were removed, his sleep got a lot better. Within just six months of undergoing the operation alongside

---

36   A. J. Yoon, S. Zaghi, S. Ha, C. S. Law, C. Guilleminault and S. Y. Liu, 'Ankyloglossia as a Risk Factor for Maxillary Hypoplasia and Soft Palate Elongation: A Functional–Morphological Study', *Orthodontics & Craniofacial Research* 20, no. 4 (2017): 237–44, https://doi.org/10.1111/ocr.12206.

37   Hye-Kyung Jung, Rok Seon Choung and Nicholas J. Talley, 'Gastroesophageal Reflux Disease and Sleep Disorders: Evidence for a Causal Link and Therapeutic Implications', *Journal of Neurogastroenterology and Motility* 16, no. 1 (2010): 22–29, https://doi.org/10.5056/jnm.2010.16.1.22.

other recommended treatments, Daniel was like a brand new kid: he was breathing and eating well with no more snoring or tantrums, and he had a big growth spurt. His improvement was measurable on the Sleep Disturbance Scale for Children,[38] where his scores almost halved from ninety-nine in March 2016 to fifty in December 2016, placing him in the normal range.

Daniel's mum wished she'd had more information when Daniel was little. His sleep is much better now, but it's hard for her to look back at 'the nightmare', as she calls it. If she'd had the information she has now before he was born, it would have made a big difference to the entire family.

There is a long list of words that parents use to describe the way kids behave when they are sleep deprived – cranky, grumpy, sleepy, clumsy, silly, crazy, fidgety (almost like Snow White's band of dwarves!)

But how do you know if these behavioural issues are caused by sleep? Daytime behaviours that result from sleep disorders can look a lot like Attention Deficit Hyperactivity Disorder (ADHD): difficulty sitting still, difficulty with concentration, focus and attention, aggression, impulsivity, interrupting, talking out of turn, hyperactivity, anxiety, trouble with literacy and more.[39] Children with ADHD also have difficulty falling sleep and staying asleep and are restless while they are asleep. In fact, snoring is common among children who have ADHD, and twenty-five per cent may have OSA.[40]

---

38 Oliviero Bruni, Salvatore Ottaviano, Vincenzo Guidetti, Manuela Romoli, Margherita Innocenzi, Flavia Cortesi and Flavia Giannotti, 'The Sleep Disturbance Scale for Children (SDSC): Construction and Validation of an Instrument to Evaluate Sleep Disturbances in Childhood and Adolescence', *Journal of Sleep Research* 5, no. 4 (1996): 251–61, https://doi.org/10.1111/j.1365-2869.1996.00251.x.

39 Dale L. Smith, David Gozal, Scott J. Hunter, Mona F. Philby, Jaeson Kaylegian and Leila Kheirandish-Gozal, 'Impact of Sleep Disordered Breathing on Behaviour among Elementary School-Aged Children: A Cross-Sectional Analysis of a Large Community-Based Sample', *European Respiratory Journal* 48, no. 6 (2016): 1631–39, https://doi.org/10.1183/13993003.00808-2016.

40 Yoo Hyun Um, Seung-Chul Hong and Jong-Hyun Jeong, 'Sleep Problems as Predictors in Attention-Deficit Hyperactivity Disorder: Causal Mechanisms, Consequences and Treatment', *Clinical Psychopharmacology and Neuroscience* 15, no. 1 (2017): 9–18, https://doi.org/10.9758/cpn.2017.15.1.9.

Kids with ADHD have problems sleeping well for many reasons, not the least of which are behaviour traits that make it difficult to settle and stay settled. Medication side effects and depression may also play a role, making it harder for them to fall asleep. Ineffective sleep, in turn, revs up behaviour further. As Dr Judith Owens says, 'Every child diagnosed with ADHD should be screened for sleep disorder. Interestingly, some of the chemicals in the brain linked to ADHD are the same involved with sleep, so the deficiency and alteration of brain chemicals necessarily leads to sleep problems.'[41]

>> all children presenting for evaluation of behavioural issues and disorders should be assessed for sleep disorders

It is Dr Owens' strong view that all children presenting for evaluation of behavioural issues and disorders should be assessed for sleep disorders.[42] This sentiment is echoed by a study at Lurie Children's Hospital Chicago and the Head and Neck Institute, Cleveland Clinic.[43]

While sleep apnoea is a serious problem, it is not our only concern. Recent studies indicate that mild sleep-disordered breathing or snoring may cause many of the same problems as OSA in children.[44] Children who snore may be at increased risk for developing attention problems and poor behaviour regulation, no matter whether the disorder is mild, moderate or severe.

Kids with runny noses and open-mouth breathing also need our attention. Depleted oxygen associated with breathing issues created by

---

41   Owens and Mindell, *Take Charge of Your Child's Sleep*.

42   Judith Owens, 'Comorbidity of Insomnia', in *14th Czech-Slovak and 19th Congress of the Czech Society for Sleep Research and Medicine*, (Prague, October 7, 2017).

43   Irina Trosman and Samuel J. Trosman, 'Cognitive and Behavioral Consequences of Sleep Disordered Breathing in Children', *Medical Sciences* 5, no. 4 (2017): 30, https://doi.org/10.3390/medsci5040030.

44   Smith et al., 'Impact of Sleep Disordered Breathing on Behaviour among Elementary School-Aged Children'.

blocked nose and throat may be an important factor causing ADHD.[45] It is therefore important that airway issues are treated as early as possible to reduce the incidence of issues like inability to sit still, and constant fidgeting.

Physical consequences of sleep problems

On a physical level, good sleep releases the right hormones, while poor sleep causes hormonal imbalance.

> >> Parents may notice their kids are not growing well, have poor appetites or are frequently sick

Parents may notice their kids are not growing well, have poor appetites or are frequently sick. Growth hormone (somatotropin) release can be missed in children who do not sleep properly. Melatonin release triggers the onset of sleep and then stimulates growth hormone, which is released three to four hours after sleep onset, so if sleep onset is delayed or sleep cycles are disrupted, growth hormone release is also delayed.[46]

'Sleep-disordered breathing, secondary to adenotonsillar hypertrophy, increases the risk of growth failure in children'.[47]

Appetite regulating hormones are also affected by sleep. The hunger and satiety hormones leptin and ghrelin play a key role in regulating the amount of food that kids consume. Imbalances in these hormone levels lead kids to craving high energy foods like sweets, biscuits and chips, followed by not realising when they are full, leading to weight gain. Obesity then contributes to poor sleep, and possibly OSA, which

45   Jiali Wu, Meizhen Gu, Shumei Chen, Wei Chen, Kun Ni, Hongming Xu and Xiaoyan Li, 'Factors Related to Pediatric Obstructive Sleep Apnea–Hypopnea Syndrome in Children with Attention Deficit Hyperactivity Disorder in Different Age Groups', Medicine 96, no. 42 (2017), https://doi.org/10.1097/md.0000000000008281.

46   Y. Takahashi, D. M. Kipnis and W. H. Daughaday, 'Growth Hormone Secretion During Sleep', Journal of Clinical Investigation 47, no. 9 (1968), https://doi.org/10.1172/jci105893.

47   Karen Bonuck, Sanjay Parikh, and Maha Bassila, 'Growth Failure and Sleep Disordered Breathing: A Review of the Literature', International Journal of Pediatric Otorhinolaryngology 70, no. 5 (2006), https://doi.org/10.1016/j.ijporl.2005.11.012.

this is borne out with other studies. Even small increments of sleep loss (as little as thirty minutes per night) can result in reduced performance on intelligence tests and affect learning in a significant way.

If a child's sleep problem is connected to disordered breathing, blood-oxygen levels drop. Any change in ideal oxygenation levels in the brain has consequences, and none are good. Low oxygenation affects every aspect of a child's health, growth and development: it worsens virtually all medical, emotional and developmental problems; it compromises a child's growth, immunity and IQ; and it impedes recovery and wellness in medically compromised patients.[52]

>> Indeed, OSA or obstructive sleep apnoea, can reduce a child's IQ by as many as ten points compared to their IQ with proper sleep

Obstructive sleep apnoea is one sleep disorder that is associated with a range of neurocognitive deficits,[53] meaning that kids are unable to focus, reason and problem solve as expected for their age. They have 'impaired attention and visual-fine motor coordination and reduction in regional grey matter.[54] This means that cells in the brain are diminishing. Research papers show that 'cortical thinning' occurs in children with sleep apnoea, and this intensifies the imperative for us all to be proactive and identify all kids with OSA.[55] Indeed, OSA or obstructive sleep apnoea, can reduce a child's IQ by as many as ten points compared to their IQ with proper

52   Owens and Mindell, *Take Charge of Your Child's Sleep.*

53   L. M. Obrien, 'Neurobehavioral Implications of Habitual Snoring in Children', *Pediatrics* 114, no. 1 (2004): 44–49, https://doi.org/10.1542/peds.114.1.44.

54   Chitra Lal, Charlie Strange and David Bachman, 'Neurocognitive Impairment in Obstructive Sleep Apnea', *Chest* 141, no. 6 (2012), https://doi.org/10.1378/chest.11-2214.

55   Paul M. Macey, Leila Kheirandish-Gozal, Janani P. Prasad, Richard A. Ma, Rajesh Kumar, Mona F. Philby and David Gozal, 'Altered Regional Brain Cortical Thickness in Pediatric Obstructive Sleep Apnea', *Frontiers in Neurology* 9 (2018), https://doi.org/10.3389/fneur.2018.00004.

sleep.[56,57] In other words, OSA can cause brain cells to decrease – not a trivial matter. One study conducted in 2006 speculated that 'untreated childhood OSA could permanently alter a developing child's cognitive potential'.[58]

Meanwhile, a study at Duke University in 2015 showed that children with attention problems in early childhood were forty per cent less likely to graduate from high school.[59] With an estimated ten per cent of children starting school with developmental delays, we can only wonder – how much of this is linked to sleep disorders?

If children get enough sleep, on the other hand, many of these problems are reversible. Bruno Giordani, professor of neurology, psychiatry, psychology and nursing at the University of Michigan, wrote, 'Regardless of intellectual level, we can expect to see some behavioural improvement along with better sleep. Once behaviour improves, attention in school improves, and emotional ability and behavioural and impulsivity control improve.'[60]

>> sleep disorders can also take their toll slowly

Long-term effects

The immediate consequences of sleep problems should be enough to convince you to take action. But sleep disorders can also take their toll slowly. By this I mean that the effects of sleep disorders build and compound over time, a bit like smoking. The first or even the thousandth cigarette won't kill you, but eventually the habit will lead

---

56 Stephen H. Sheldon, Richard Ferber, Meir H. Kryger and David Gozal, *Principles and Practice of Pediatric Sleep Medicine*, (London: Elsevier Saunders, 2014).

57 Matt Wood, 'The Deep Impact of Childhood Sleep Apnea', University of Chicago Medicine, posted on March 1, 2012, https://sciencelife.uchospitals.edu/2012/03/01/the-deep-impact-of-childhood-sleep-apnea.

58 Halbower et al., 'Childhood Obstructive Sleep Apnea Associates with Neuropsychological Deficits and Neuronal Brain Injury'.

59 David L. Rabiner, Jennifer Godwin and Kenneth A. Dodge, 'Predicting Academic Achievement and Attainment: The Contribution of Early Academic Skills, Attention Difficulties, and Social Competence', *School Psychology Review* 45, no. 2 (2016): 250–67, https://doi.org/10.17105/spr45-2.250-267.

60 'Even Children with Higher IQs Behave Better When Their Sleep Apnea Is Fixed', University of Michigan, January 8, 2016, http://ihpi.umich.edu/news/even-children-higher-iqs-behave-better-when-their-sleep-apnea-fixed.

to an earlier death as it erodes your lung capacity, deprives the brain of oxygen and poisons your system. Similarly, with some forms of skin cancer, the first exposure to high-UV sun may not give you melanoma, but repeated exposure will leave you highly susceptible. These facts are well known and largely accepted in Australia, which has launched successful health campaigns to educate everyone on the dangers of smoking and high-UV sun exposure.

>> Professor Karen Bonuck demonstrated that behaviour difficulties at seven years and special education at eight years were linked to having had sleep problems prior to five years of age

Sleep disorders are similar. Prolonged exposure to poor sleep quality, sleep deprivation and fragmentation means children experience ongoing behavioural, physical and emotional consequences that then compound over time. In addition, they are at risk of developing the associated health issues such as increased blood pressure and cardiac problems. Professor Karen Bonuck demonstrated that behaviour difficulties at seven years and special education at eight years were linked to having had sleep problems prior to five years of age.[61] Furthermore, both SDB and short sleep duration significantly and independently increase children's odds of becoming overweight.[62]

Dr Kate Williams from Queensland University of Technology analysed the sleep behaviour of 2,800 children born in 2004 until they reached six to seven years of age in the landmark study, *Growing up in Australia: The Longitudinal Study of Australian Children*. She found that, while seventy

61   Karen Bonuck, 'Pediatric Sleep Disorders and Special Educational Need at 8 Years: A Population-Based Cohort Study', *Pediatrics* 130, no. 4 (2012), https://doi.org/10.1542/peds.2012-0392d.
62   Karen Bonuck, Ronald D. Chervin and Laura D. Howe, 'Sleep-Disordered Breathing, Sleep Duration, and Childhood Overweight: A Longitudinal Cohort Study', *The Journal of Pediatrics* 166, no. 3 (2015), https://doi.org/10.1016/j.jpeds.2014.11.001.

per cent of children were regulating their own sleep by five years of age, the remaining thirty per cent might find their lack of regulation developmentally detrimental over time.[63]

Consequently, it's vital to get children's sleep behaviours right by the time they turn five. 'If these sleep issues aren't resolved by the time children are five years old, then they are at risk of poorer adjustment to school,' Williams said. This has been backed by other studies.[64] Simply getting children to bed earlier than 9:30pm improves behaviour,[65] and children who soothe themselves back to sleep from an early age adjust to school more easily than those who don't.[66,67] Helping parents get the sleep formula right when kids are young can make a big difference to everyone. Parents need a good support network.

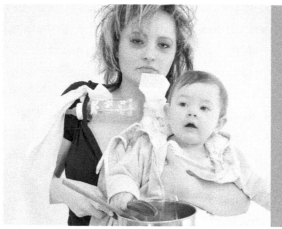

Helping parents get the sleep formula right when kids are young can make a big difference to everyone. Parents need a good support network.

63   'Growing Up in Australia: The Longitudinal Study of Australian Children', Australian Institute of Family Studies, http://www.growingupinaustralia.gov.au/.

64   Rabiner, Godwin and Dodge, 'Predicting Academic Achievement and Attainment: The Contribution of Early Academic Skills, Attention Difficulties, and Social Competence'.

65   'News – Get Sleep Sorted By Age 5 To Help Children Settle At School', Queensland University of Technology, Interview with Dr Kate Williams, March 9, 2016, https://www.qut.edu.au/news?news-id=102587.

66   Matthew Gray and Diana Smart, 'Growing Up in Australia: The Longitudinal Study of Australian Children: A Valuable New Data Source for Economists', *Australian Economic Review* 42, no. 3 (2009): 367–76, https://doi.org/10.1111/j.1467-8462.2009.00555.x.

67   Kate E. Williams, Jan M. Nicholson, Sue Walker and Donna Berthelsen, 'Early Childhood Profiles of Sleep Problems and Self-Regulation Predict Later School Adjustment', *British Journal of Educational Psychology* 86, no. 2 (2016): 331–50, https://doi.org/10.1111/bjep.12109.

Sleep deprivation in kids with special needs

'Some days I am so tired that I could just cry. Actually, some days I am so tired that I do cry. But our own exhaustion is not even the worst part. The hardest part is watching our little man struggle through his tired haze.'[68] These words from Jessica Sylfest, talking about her four-year-old autistic son in *The Huffington Post*, hit at the heart of a major struggle for parents with special needs children – the ongoing exhaustion of it all.

Kids with special needs are particularly susceptible to sleep problems. As Dr Judith Owens points out, 'There's a very high prevalence of insomnia in autism spectrum disorders – thirty-four to eighty-nine per cent of kids with autism spectrum disorders also have sleep disorders. Early intervention is critical for caregivers with these kids, given the demands of the day, and parents' sleep disturbance on top of it.'[69]

Due to the nature of their difficulties, many kids with disabilities may need to spend time in hospital for treatments and surgeries. This can be very challenging because hospitals are noisy, stressful places for children and their families, and it's hard to sleep. Even the best sleepers have trouble drifting off or staying asleep in a hospital; being woken up multiple times a night to have vitals checked disrupts their sleep pattern and leads to more sleep problems when they come home. Common medications also have side effects that can complicate sleep efficacy.[70]

At home, autistic children, or those with varying degrees of developmental delay, often have trouble settling into sleep and back to sleep if they wake. Due to their susceptibility to sensory overload, these kids can become wired and anxious, unable to wind down and self-soothe before bed. It can take up to two or three hours for them to fall asleep after bedtime. If they go to sleep late or wake early, they are consistently

---

68   Jessica Sylfest, 'The Truth About Autism and Sleep', Huffington Post, last modified January 18, 2017, https://www.huffingtonpost.com/entry/587f775ce4b0474ad4874f2f.
69   Owens and Mindell, *Take Charge of Your Child's Sleep*.
70   Ibid.

not getting enough sleep, and the quality of the sleep they *do* get is disrupted by night waking. This could be due to habit, waking in transition between sleep cycles or remaining in light sleep throughout the night.

This all then exacerbates the cycle of overwhelm. After a night of poor sleep, the next day is then pre-set for more 'wired but tired' behaviour and anxiety. And the cycle repeats itself. As any family in this sleep-fog, wired-tired cycle will tell you, it is not a fun place to be.

Take Wendy, an eight-year-old girl with Down syndrome who suffered from everything – severe diarrhoea, the flu, pneumonia. She was constantly sick, week in and week out, and had a very slow growth rate. She had no energy and didn't want to get out of bed. At the same time, her parents would find her sitting up in bed at night, trying to catch her breath.

When she was hospitalised for pneumonia, it was discovered that she was suffering from OSA, which affects at least fifty per cent of children with Down syndrome. Further investigation found she had enlarged tonsils and adenoids blocking her already small airways.

For Wendy, when she lay down to sleep and moved into sleep phases where deeper muscle relaxation occurred, there was airway obstruction and her breathing stopped several times an hour. Not only that, kids with Down syndrome have anatomy that predisposes them to OSA – they usually have a small narrow upper jaw, which means there's not enough room for the tongue in the mouth, and the tongue looks too big. Restricted space in the mouth makes the airway even more crowded and vulnerable to airway obstruction, so when tonsils and adenoids are enlarged, the airway becomes really crowded.

Once Wendy's adenoids were removed, her sleep improved. She was less sleepy and grumpy during the day, which made living with Wendy a lot easier. She had a growth spurt, became a much happier kid with a lot more energy, and contracted colds and tummy bugs less frequently. But some symptoms remained.

We noticed that although her sleep was much better, she continued to have restless sleep, noisy breathing and groggy waking in the mornings. Even though the OSA was resolved, Wendy still had a milder version of obstructed breathing. Kids with Down syndrome also have low-tone muscles, and this was a plausible explanation for the ongoing airway issue. She also continued to have middle ear fluid and occasional chesty coughing after eating meals – additional signs that the upper airway was not working perfectly and that ongoing monitoring was important.

Kids with disabilities, chronic medical conditions like Down syndrome, joint laxity (such as Ehlers-Danlos syndrome) and craniofacial syndromes (such as Pierre Robin, Crouzon, Apert, Prader-Willi and Pfeiffer syndromes) are airway challenged due to the shape, size and position of the bones that make up the head and face.[71] These conditions are associated with smaller or constricted upper airways such as small or uneven nasal passages, which may lead to habitual mouth breathing. This then leads to disruption of oxygen to the brain and is on the spectrum of sleep-disordered breathing.[72] Weak, low-tone muscles in the upper airway also make kids more susceptible to upper airway collapse during sleep.

This is where myofunctional training (See Chapter 5) became vital for Wendy. Myofunctional programs improve the muscle systems of the mouth, face and throat and improve their airway, along with retraining breathing habits. When the upper throat muscles are working at their best, it can even help kids with clearing fluid from the middle ears. That's exactly what we did with Wendy. Over time, with myofunctional therapy, Wendy no longer needed grommets. She was able to get quiet, uninterrupted sleep, and today she is a happy kid, doing all the things young girls love to do – riding ponies, growing vegies in her own vegie patch and dancing – all while she is breathing, eating and sleeping well.

71   Christian Guilleminault and Yu-Shu Huang, 'From Oral Facial Dysfunction to Dysmorphism and the Onset Of Pediatric OSA', *Sleep Medicine Reviews*, 2017, https://doi.org/:10.1016/j.smrv.2017.06.008.

72   Esfandiar Niaki, Javad Chalipa, and Elahe Taghipoor, 'Evaluation of Oxygen Saturation by Pulse-Oximetry in Mouth Breathing Patients', *Acta Medica Iranica* 48, no. 1 (15 February 2010).

>> Good sleep is essential to help us grow and develop properly, regulate our body functions in a healthy way and protect us from illness. Poor or adequate sleep is not an option

It's time to act

Countless studies demonstrate the importance of sleep. If you read nothing else in this book, it's essential you recognise that *good sleep matters a lot*. Good sleep is a requirement for the brain to maintain and repair tissues and replenish hormones. Good sleep is essential to help us grow and develop properly, regulate our body functions in a healthy way and protect us from illness. Poor or adequate sleep is not an option.

But what does this 'good sleep' actually look like, and how can you tell if your child is suffering from disordered sleep or a sleep disorder? In the same way lifeguards know how to pick a safe spot to swim and direct beachgoers to swim between the flags, to be a lifeguard of your children's sleep you need to be able to tell good sleep from sleep problems so you will be able to encourage your children in the right direction. Continue to Chapter 2, where I discuss the essential processes that take place during good sleep, as well as outlining some of the most common sleep disorders in kids.

CHAPTER TWO

Understanding sleep problems

Let's just start by saying that a lot of kids have sleep problems.

Here are some numbers to ponder. Studies show that twenty to thirty per cent of children have significant bedtime problems or night waking, and in most cases, these have behavioural causes and solutions. Behavioural sleep problems are found in all age groups. This means behaviours like refusal, resistance or revving up at bedtime.

>> Developmental changes and phases can disrupt sleep patterns and routines. During these times, babies need more reassurance and comforting

For infants and toddlers, night wakings are one of the most common sleep problems; twenty-five to fifty per cent of children over the age of six months continue to awaken during the night. There are developmental phases and changes that can help to explain night waking for littlies, including sleep regression, separation anxiety and teething, which can disrupt sleep patterns and routines. During these times, babies need more reassurance and comforting. Bedtime resistance is found in ten to fifteen per cent of toddlers. For preschool-aged children, fifteen to thirty per cent have difficulties falling asleep or wake during the night. For school-aged children, although previously thought to be rare, surveys suggest that sleep problems are present in twenty-five to forty per cent of four- to ten-year-old children. Fifteen per cent of these children have bedtime resistance and almost eleven per cent have sleep-related anxiety

>> Sleep disorders require a medical diagnosis. Disordered sleep, in contrast, refers to situations where kids' sleep is disrupted for other reasons, like a poor routine, a poor sleep environment or emotional disturbances

(that is, 'conditioned' insomnia).[73] These behavioural sleep problems often mean kids don't get to bed at the ideal time, or get enough sleep. And did you know that sleep deprived kids are twice as likely to break the rules?[74]

Sleep disorders require a medical diagnosis. The true percentage is difficult to determine, however, five to ten per cent of children snore regularly,[75] two to four per cent have obstructive sleep apnoea,[76] and others experience variations of upper airway obstruction such as upper airway resistance syndrome or other diagnosable sleep disorders like restless leg syndrome.[77] Some have milder sleep disturbances from issues such as mouth breathing. Disordered sleep, in contrast, refers to situations where kids' sleep is disrupted for other reasons, like a poor routine, a poor sleep environment or emotional disturbances.

Yet sleep myths abound.

When I first started talking to parents about sleep about five years ago, I heard all sorts of beliefs, myths and wives' tales that helped me understand parents' belief systems around sleep for children.

Just some of these include:

73 Judith A. Owens and Ronald D. Chervin, 'Behavioral Sleep Problems in Children', UpToDate, last updated February 23, 2017, https://www.uptodate.com/contents/behavioral-sleep-problems-in-children.

74 Scott Burgess, presentation, *AAOM Inc Symposium Day* (Coolangatta, February 17, 2018).

75 Smith et al., 'Impact of Sleep Disordered Breathing on Behaviour among Elementary School-Aged Children'.

76 Ibid.

77 Michael Gelb and Howard Hindin, *GASP Airway Health: The Hidden Path to Wellness,* (CreateSpace Independent Publishing Platform, 2016).

- 'He'll grow out of it.'
- 'It's just the way she is – so sweet.'
- 'Oh, he snores all the time, but just snores quietly.'
- 'Ha ha – she snores just like her dad.'
- 'Ear infections and getting sick; it's normal.'
- 'How cute – he sleeps in snail position.'
- 'He wakes up with his head at the wrong end of the bed … how precious.'
- 'The bed always looks like a cyclone hit it.'
- 'Oh yes, I can hear her breathe. At least I know she's alive.'
- 'If he's snoring loudly I know he's in a deep sleep.'
- 'Most kids wet the bed; she just took a long time to grow out of it.'
- 'He sounds like a freight train when he grinds his teeth. Lucky he's at the other end of the house.'
- 'She's just like her father; she wakes all the time.'
- 'My grandma snores and she's just fine.'
- 'Being sleepless – that's just part of being a parent!'

>> It's a myth that some children don't need much sleep

Such ideas encourage parents not to worry about their child's symptoms, which means they don't get treated, and kids don't get the sleep they need.

It's time that such beliefs and sleep myths are debunked. As Dr Judith Owens says, 'It's a myth that some children don't need much sleep. It's true that most children can't tell you when they are tired and, even if they knew they were tired, they are unlikely to own up. But *all* children need sleep, and the right amount. They don't adapt or adjust or develop resilience to poor sleep or sleep deprivation; they simply don't thrive, don't grow and don't learn as well.'[78]

Sadly, misdirected beliefs about sleep are not limited to parents. I have had patients whose parents have asked their GP or specialist about signs and symptoms they were noticing, only to be assured that it is just a

78 Owens and Mindell, *Take Charge of Your Child's Sleep*.

phase and that their child will grow out of it. Yet after speaking with parents about the signs and symptoms of sleep disorders, the common responses are: 'I wish I'd known that before', 'I just thought it would pass', 'I assumed nothing could be done', or 'I didn't realise it was a problem'.

Consequently, it's crucial that you, as a parent, become the 'first responder' to your child's sleep issues rather than waiting for someone else to take on that role. This may require re-examining your own assumptions and beliefs about sleep.

You are the person with the most commitment to your child's welfare and the greatest insight into their real sleep habits. In your role as a lifeguard, understanding the difference between good sleep and bad sleep will help you better understand if there's a problem. Early recognition means early treatment is possible, and the earlier you tackle these issues, the better.

>> For some of us, poor sleep goes on so long that it becomes the new normal

What is good sleep?

We all know the feeling of poor sleep and not waking well. We know its lingering effects throughout the day. However, many people don't know what *good* sleep is. For some of us, poor sleep goes on so long that it becomes the new normal.

Recently I was in a clinical session with an eight-year-old girl, and she was calm, still and attentive for the first time ever. I also learnt that, for the first time ever, she had had *three consecutive nights* of uninterrupted quiet sleep, the right amount for her age (ten to eleven hours). Her mum told me, emotionally, 'Jillian has been wired and sleepless for so long, I just thought it was normal.'

So, what is good sleep? Good sleep is silent, uninterrupted sleep, for the recommended number of hours according to age, which results in waking refreshed. In the following pages, I'll share the basics of how sleep works and what to expect when you and your kids are sleeping well.

The types and stages of sleep

There are two types of sleep: rapid eye movement (REM) and non-rapid eye movement (non-REM) sleep.

Within non-REM, there are four stages of sleep. Stages 1 and 2 are light sleep, while stages 3 and 4 (usually seen as a combined phase) are deep sleep. In each of these stages there is different brain and body activity, meaning your brain waves, breathing and heart rate all change.

- **Stage 1:** This stage, occurring between wakefulness and sleep, usually takes five per cent of your total sleep time. During this stage, the heart rate slows down, and sleep is very light and easily disrupted.

- **Stage 2:** This stage is the longest sleep phase, being forty-five to fifty per cent of your total sleep time. In stage 2, all your muscles start to relax, including your throat muscles, which is why snoring may occur, and responses to outside stimuli are suppressed. This stage helps the brain consolidate information and learnings from the day, including the mastery of motor or physical skills.

- **Stage 3:** This stage, when combined with stage 4, takes twenty-five per cent of your total sleep time. It is the deepest phase of sleep, during which your temperature, heart rate and breathing rate are all at their lowest. Your brain and body further relax and are even less responsive to the outside world. This is the stage where parasomnias and bed-wetting can occur. It is also when declarative memory (long-term memory for facts, previous experiences, world knowledge and new concepts) consolidates and newly learnt memories are reactivated.

- **Stage 4:** During this stage your brain activity is at its lowest, and deepest sleep occurs. Deep sleep in stages 3 and 4 allows the release of hormones related to growing and tissue repair, which is critical for waking refreshed.

There's a lot going

NON-REM SLEEP

STAGE 1

Eyes move slowly, heart rate and muscle activity slows, can have sudden movements or leg jerks, light sleep easily roused by light, sound or touch

Transition phase from awake to deeper sleep, brain is preparing for stage 2

Overstimulation or anxiety can prevent entry to the next phase of sleep, cause delayed sleep times

STAGE 2

Eye movement stops, temperature begins to drop and heart rate slows, muscles relax and this can lead to snoring, less likelihood of waking with light, sound or touch

Consolidation of learning from the day just gone, including; physical and coordination skills

Sleep disordered breathing can disturb this phase and interrupt entry to deeper phases of sleep

STAGE 3

Temperature heart rate and breathing are very low, deep slow wave sleep occurs, brain activity slows, deep slow wave sleep occurs, growth and tissue repair

Declarative memory consolidation, release of hormones for growth and tissue repair, refreshes ready for new learning next day

Bedwetting and/or parasomnias when the cycle is disturbed

STAGE 4

Brain activity is at the absolute lowest, very difficult to rouse, deepest slow wave sleep, no eye movement, no muscle activity, growth and tissue repair

Declarative memory consolidation, release of hormones for growth and tissue repair, refreshes ready for new learning next day

Parasomnias and or night terrors

 What is happening in the body

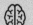 What is happening in the brain

 What can go wrong

on during sleep

To wake fully refreshed and ready for the day, you need to pass through all 4 stages and REM sleep every night, multiple times, for the recommended hours of sleep.

The full non-REM cycle takes about ninety minutes in adults. The usual sleep cycle progresses through stages 1, 2, 3 and 4, then back to stage 2, and then REM sleep kicks in. Between each full sleep cycle there's a brief awakening, but most people are unaware of this as it only lasts seconds before they drift into another sleep cycle.

REM sleep occurs in stages, starting with a ten-minute period of REM sleep and increasing throughout the night, with the final REM stage lasting up to an hour. A series of four or five sleep cycles of non-REM and REM sleep occur every night. The first cycle is about ninety minutes, and successive cycles last from 100 to 120 minutes. However, babies and toddlers will cycle through non-REM stages to REM more often, depending on the number of hours they sleep.

>> During REM sleep, dreaming occurs, which is vital for enhancing memory and dealing with traumatic events

During REM sleep, dreaming occurs, which is vital for enhancing memory and dealing with traumatic events. The body is 'paralysed' during this stage, except for the breathing muscles – a feature that stops us from acting out vivid dreams. However, there is still a lot of electrical and chemical activity taking place in your brain, including the removal of toxins, the release of hormones and other chemical exchanges. Even your dreams are helping you to manage and solve problems, along with consolidating emotional memory.

Procedural and spatial memory are also created during REM. Procedural memory recalls routine actions, tasks and skills like brushing teeth and getting dressed, while spatial memory recalls how things are laid out in space, like how to get to the shops from your home, or how to go to the back door of your house.

The brain's oxygen consumption and energy consumption is very high during REM – even higher than when awake and working on a complex

>> Lack of REM impairs our ability to learn complex tasks, especially during early childhood

problem. Your breathing rate increases, along with your heart rate and blood pressure, to near waking levels. Core temperature is not well regulated during the paralysed muscle state of REM.

We need to experience all stages of non-REM and REM sleep to have optimal brain and body restoration. Lack of REM impairs our ability to learn complex tasks, especially during early childhood. Waking naturally after four, five or more full sleep cycles (depending on age) is the best way to ensure that you have had just the right amount of sleep.

What happens in REM sleep DREAM LAND

 Blood pressure breathing & heart rate increases to almost awake levels, but all muscles are 'paralysed'. There is high energy and oxygen consumption, removals of toxins and waste from the brain, & hormone release

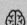 Enhances memory (procedural and spatial), deal with trauma, consolidate learning of complex tasks e.g. speech, bike riding, walking, etc

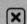 Miss out on essential REM due to early waking or sleep disruption, sleep cycles are disrupted by sleep disorder, sleep paralysis (rare)

 What is happening in the body

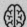 What is happening in the brain

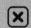 What can go wrong

To wake fully refreshed and ready for the day, you need to pass through all 4 stages and REM sleep every night, multiple times, for the recommended hours of sleep.

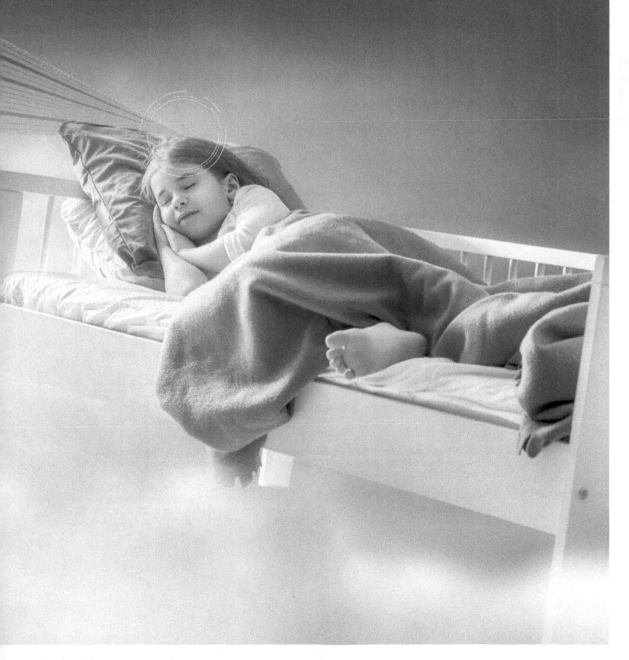

The essential function
of dreams

SLEEP AND THE MAGIC OF YOUR BRAIN[79]

Scientists used to think that the brain went to sleep when we slept. In fact, the opposite is true. New science paints a very different picture about what the brain gets up to during sleep, and it's akin to magic. It's called glymphatics.[80]

This process was unknown until recently, when researchers discovered 'a giant nocturnal distribution network' that parallels the extensive blood system in our brain. The system is a fluid filled channel that literally opens up at night once we are asleep. Brain cells called glial cells shrink, allowing the channel system to open up and fill with cerebro-spinal fluid. Many chemical and hormonal transactions occur between the brain cells and fluid. These exchanges occur throughout the phases of sleep and are essential to good brain health.

During his TED talk 'One more reason to get a good night's sleep', neuroscientist Jeff Iliff describes the glymphatic system as 'an elegant and clever design solution to some of the brain's most basic needs: the continuous supply of nutrients, distributing lipids and glucose within the brain, clearing waste, and regulating essential hormones and neuropeptides, which control growth, immunity, appetite, sugar cravings and more. It is a specialised network of plumbing that organises and facilitates this process. The plumbing system means every tiny corner of the brain can be

79   Nadia Aalling Jessen, Anne Sofie Finmann Munk, Iben Lundgaard and Maiken Nedergaard, 'The Glymphatic System: A Beginner's Guide', *Neurochemical Research* 40, no. 12 (2015), https://doi.org/10.1007/s11064-015-1581-6.

80   J. J. Iliff, M. Wang, Y. Liao, B. A. Plogg, W. Peng, G. A. Gundersen, H. Benveniste, G. E. Vates, R. Deane, S. A. Goldman, E. A. Nagelhus and M. Nedergaard, 'A Paravascular Pathway Facilitates CSF Flow through the Brain Parenchyma and the Clearance of Interstitial Solutes, Including Amyloid β', *Science Translational Medicine* 4, no. 147 (2012), https://doi.org/10.1126/scitranslmed.3003748.

reached. But the whole thing only happens in the sleeping brain. It is this feature that may have made its discovery so difficult.'[81]

One aspect of the waste clearance allows the rapid removal of a toxic waste product in the brain called amyloid-beta, which is linked to Alzheimer's. Worsening sleep quality and sleep duration are associated with a greater amount of amyloid-beta building up in the brain, which is why poor glymphatic function is thought to contribute to pathology in neurodegenerative disorders like Alzheimer's and Parkinson's, and to traumatic brain injury and stroke.

Iliff likens the glymphatic system to house cleaning. In our homes, when the cleaning is not done properly on a regular basis, things get shabby and go downhill. When it comes to cleaning the brain, if brain processing and memory consolidation is not happening, you can't be at your best. The process can only occur fully when all stages of sleep are expressed three, four, five (or more with babies) times a night.

The implication is that you need to go through all sleep cycles, including all the phases of REM and non-REM sleep, every night, for the brain 'glymphatics' to complete essential 'cleaning' and preparation for the following day. Good sleep matters a lot.

>> you need to go through all sleep cycles, including all the phases of REM and non-REM sleep, every night, for the brain 'glymphatics' to complete essential 'cleaning' and preparation for the following day

81   Jeff Iliff, 'One More Reason to Get a Good Night's Sleep', Filmed September 2014 at TEDMED 2014, TED video, https://www.ted.com/talks/jeff_iliff_one_more_reason_to_get_a_good_night_s_sleep.

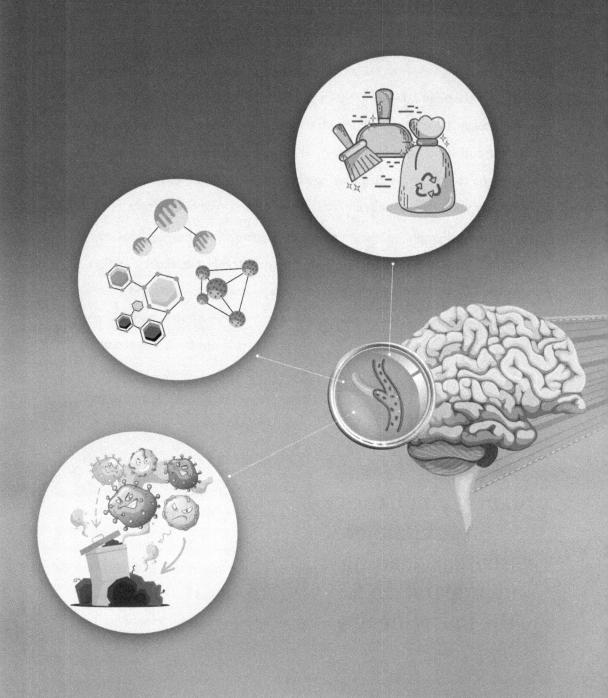

The busy brain during sleep

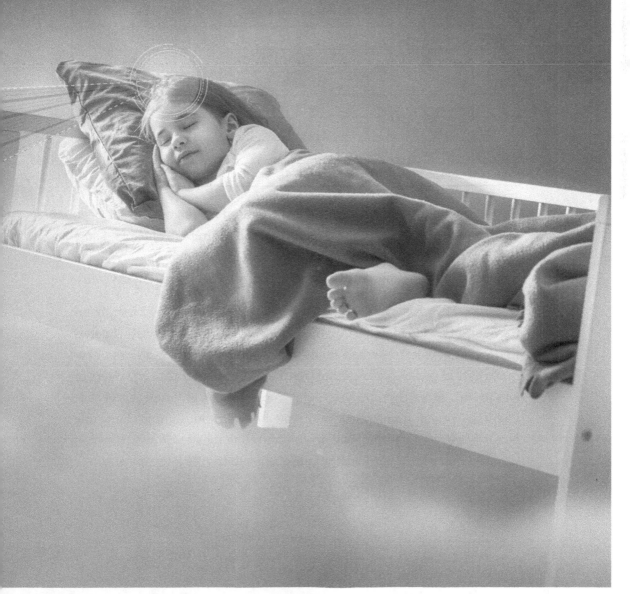

How much sleep do you need?

With the different sleep stages in mind, how much sleep do you and your kids need in order to experience the most benefits?

This varies by age, with younger children needing more sleep and adults needing less, and can vary by individual.

However, the following table provides a guide and is based on the American Academy of Sleep Medicine guidelines, which are grounded in up to date scientific research:

	Number of hours sleep	Percent of day[1]
Newborns: 0–3 months	14–17	58–71%
Infants: 4–2 months	12–16	50–67%
Toddlers: 1–2 years	11–14	45–58%
Preschoolers: 3–5 years	10–13	42–54%
Children: 6–12 years	9–12	37.5–50%
Teenagers: 13–18 years	8–10	33–42%
Adults: 18+	7–9	29–37.5%

As you see from the numbers, there is variation for the amount of sleep needed at each age group, and this depends on a number of factors. Some common ones include sleep drive, which builds through the day and is dependent on nap times and daily activities, and also circadian rhythms.

Circadian rhythms usually develop within six months after birth, helping babies to sleep more during the night-time. Circadian rhythms determine daytime alertness and night-time sleepiness. Each person's circadian rhythm varies, determining whether they are natural early risers or late to bed. These rhythms are highly dependent on environmental cues like light, sound, atmosphere and activity levels, but light is the prime factor because of its influence on the hormone melatonin which, when released in the brain as daylight fades, helps to trigger sleep onset.

Some individuals have a rare genetic condition that means they truly need less sleep.[82] However, only one to three per cent of the population can get by on just six hours every night. The explanation for those who need less sleep lies in gene expression.[83] It is not something we can train ourselves to need less of.

>> too little or too much both have their down sides, whereas just right is literally just right, according to the recommended sleep hours for your age

Richard Wiseman talks about the Goldilocks principle when it comes to getting the correct number of hours of sleep: too little or too much both have their down sides, whereas just right is literally just right, according to the recommended sleep hours for your age.[84] Naturally, if you are unwell, healing from an injury or growing, your body may need more sleep. Beyond this, however, it's best to stick with 'just right'. While it's hard to imagine that too much sleep could harm you, it may be a sign of an underlying medical condition and is associated with increased risk of developing medical conditions like diabetes, depression, respiratory and heart problems.

82 Arianna S. Huffington, *The Sleep Revolution: Transforming Your Life, One Night at a Time* (New York: Harmony, 2016).

83 Y. He, C. R. Jones, N. Fujiki, Y. Xu, B. Guo, J. L. Holder, M. J. Rossner, S. Nishino and Y. H. Fu, 'The Transcriptional Repressor DEC2 Regulates Sleep Length in Mammals', *Science* 325, no. 5942 (2009), https://doi.org/10.1126/science.1174443.

84 Wiseman, *Night School: The Life-Changing Science of Sleep.*

The Stages

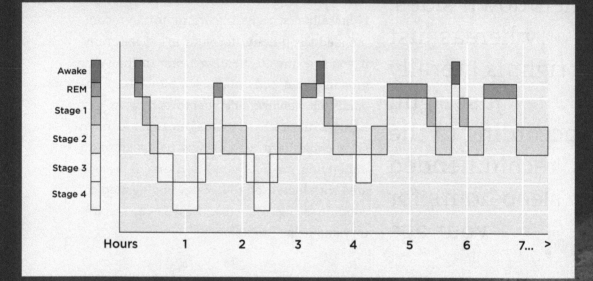

Awake
REM
Stage 1
Stage 2
Stage 3
Stage 4

Hours   1   2   3   4   5   6   7... >

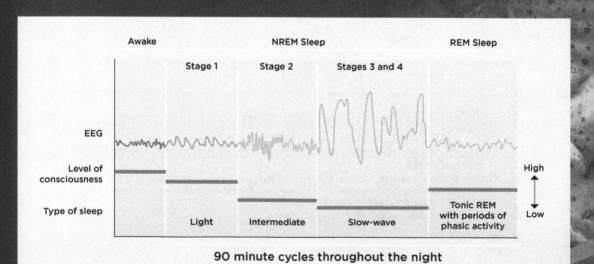

Awake   NREM Sleep   REM Sleep

Stage 1   Stage 2   Stages 3 and 4

EEG

Level of
consciousness

High

Type of sleep

Low

Light   Intermediate   Slow-wave   Tonic REM
with periods of
phasic activity

90 minute cycles throughout the night

# of Sleep

The sleep formula:
silent, uninterrupted sleep
for the recommended number
of hours each night, and waking
refreshed and ready for the day.

The good sleep formula

When you put these considerations together, the formula for good sleep is fairly simple:

RIGHT **QUALITY** + RIGHT **QUANTITY** = **GOOD SLEEP**.

» Good sleep means quiet, uninterrupted sleep for the recommended number of hours, and waking refreshed

The quality and quantity of your sleep are inseparable. If you get quality sleep but not enough of it, brain rejuvenation is incomplete. If you get enough sleep but it is of a poor quality (in other words, you aren't cycling through the different stages effectively or enough), brain rejuvenation is incomplete.

Remember? Good sleep means quiet, uninterrupted sleep for the recommended number of hours, and waking refreshed. If you get the right formula, you feel happier, calmer, less hungry, more energetic and less inclined to need a boost from that energy drink, caffeine hit or sugary food. Your thinking skills are sharp, you are more creative, you have more physical energy and you have better immunity.

Unfortunately, sleep disorders and disordered sleep disrupt both the quality and quantity of sleep.

To be a good sleeper you need

Right **Quality** of sleep: silent, uninterrupted, still, wake refreshed

Right **Quantity** of sleep: hours in a 24 hour period

Any interruptions to quality and quantity disturb critical processes in the brain. (Learn more about sleep and the brain on pages 54 and 55)

The important concept is *consistency*. It isn't enough to get one night of good sleep – you and your kids should be experiencing good sleep *every night*. Why get good sleep? Consistently achieving the good sleep formula sets the scene for you and your children to be at your best; physically, mentally, socially and emotionally.

>> **These days we are all are over-scheduled, over-committed, overtired and over-extended, which leads many of us to believe we can train ourselves to do more on less sleep**

These days we are all are over-scheduled, over-committed, overtired and over-extended, which leads many of us to believe we can train ourselves to do more on less sleep. It is common to hear people say they can catch up on lost sleep, but the truth is that you can't. The Goldilocks principle dictates that you need a consistent amount of sleep. It is not advised to attempt a catch up by sleeping in on weekends, as this disrupts the routine for the days following, which in turn disrupts the brain's associations with routine and environment that usually trigger sleep. Each time you or your kids lose sleep or experience poor sleep, you create a debt that cannot be 'caught up', or at least, research hasn't figured out how that may be able to happen.

As I touched on last chapter, the effects of sleep problems can be slow. After one night of poor quality sleep you may feel groggy and not at your best. However, after many nights of sleep problems like sleep-disordered breathing, your body may be in a developing state of inflammation or decline that eventually lead to conditions like high blood pressure, cardiac disorders, metabolic disorders, obesity, depression and cancer.[85]

---

85   Nieto et al., 'Sleep-Disordered Breathing and Cancer Mortality'.

What is bad sleep?

Now that we've looked at good sleep, what is *bad* sleep?

Bad sleep runs along a continuum, but pretty much anything that interrupts the quantity, quality and consistency of your sleep is somewhere on the bad scale, no matter how mild. Mild difficulties may be something you feel you can just put up with, but they have a hidden cost, leading to a build-up of sleep debt over time.

There are over ninety different sleep disorders. While it's not possible to go into all of them in depth, the rest of this chapter focuses on covering some of the more common disorders. It is critical to have sleep disorders properly diagnosed and treated by medical experts. I've provided descriptions here to help you identify red flags in your child's sleep (or your own) so that you'll know when to seek help.

A guide to common sleep disorders

INSOMNIA

Insomnia is by far the most common sleep disorder. It leads to sleep disruption, fragmentation and poor sleep quality because of difficulty falling asleep, waking in the middle of the night and having trouble getting back to sleep, or waking earlier in the morning than planned.

Insomniacs wake unrefreshed, are excessively sleepy during the day, and have all the usual symptoms of poor sleep including a lack of energy, being tired but wired, poor concentration, moodiness, poor memory, relationship difficulties and depression. They are more prone to accidents – with adults this could be work or car accidents, while with kids it could be clumsiness, falls and bumps.

SLEEP-DISORDERED BREATHING (SDB)

Sleep-disordered breathing (SDB) is a general term for breathing difficulties occurring during sleep. SDB disrupts the normal transitions through sleep cycles, preventing kids from moving into or staying in the restorative phases of deep sleep. SDB is the second most common sleep disorder.

When a child's breathing is disrupted during sleep, the body perceives this as a choking phenomenon. Narrowing of the airway, caused by factors like relaxed airway muscles or poor sleep position, can lead to flow limitation where the body has to work harder just to breathe, and the size of the breath is not ideal. In this situation, heart rate increases, blood pressure rises, the brain is aroused, sleep phases are interrupted and critical brain processes are disrupted. Oxygen levels in the blood can also drop, which impacts both brain and body.

If 'work of breath' escalates to breath hold moments, as happens in sleep apnoea, breath stoppages may last for ten seconds or more. These repeated interruptions to breathing place stress on the body systems, so much so that their effects have been likened to those from the effort of breathing while altitude climbing on Mount Everest.

Disorders on the SDB spectrum include:

- **Obstructive sleep apnoea (OSA):** OSA is a condition involving repeated episodes of partial or complete blockage of the airway during sleep. These intermittent drops in oxygen lead to sleep fragmentation and poor quality sleep. When breathing stops for ten seconds or more, one to five times per hour, it is classified as mild OSA. Five to ten times per hour means moderate OSA, and more than ten times per hour equals severe OSA. OSA is a life-threatening disorder and has catastrophic effects: 'The consequences of OSA are isolation, depression, memory loss, hyperactivity, inattention, excessive daytime sleepiness, poor school performance and health challenges like elevated blood pressure. It leads to ADHD-like behaviour, and kids with OSA have less empathy. They may be bullies or they may be bullied. Their quality of life is really poor.'[86,87] Fortunately, when you

86   Kheirandish-Gozal, 'Morbidity of OSA in Children'.
87   Macey et al., 'Altered Regional Brain Cortical Thickness in Pediatric Obstructive Sleep Apnea'.

fix the OSA, behaviour can improve very quickly. Adenotonsillectomy (removal of tonsils and adenoids) is the most common treatment for OSA. However, while it may reduce the most severe clinical symptoms, there may be residual difficulties that still fall under the SDB category, so it's important to check for these. Sadly, many kids with OSA are misdiagnosed, or a diagnosis is missed altogether.

- **Snoring**: Snoring occurs when air is squeezed through an obstruction or narrowing in the airway. The obstruction can occur along a point in the upper airway, most commonly at the back of the nose or tongue. Relaxation of the throat muscles makes the airway too narrow, leading to vibrations in the throat muscles and soft palate or back of the tongue as air passes through. This creates noisy breathing or snoring. Approximately ten per cent of children snore regularly, with many parents assuming that snoring means their child is in a deep sleep. Unfortunately, very few parents are aware of how serious snoring is (even quiet snoring), as it reduces the level of oxygen that can reach the lungs, blood stream and brain. It leads to sleep arousals and fragmentation and is more common when sleeping on your back.

- **Upper airway resistance syndrome (UARS)**: UARS is a sleep disorder caused by resistance to breathing during sleep, usually caused by a physical narrowing of the airway. UARS can cause symptoms similar to those found in OSA, including excessive daytime sleepiness and fatigue. Resistance to breathing occurs in the upper airway, leading to repeated arousals, which are typically short, one to three breaths in duration, and are not detected in the usual sleep study. Measurement of these requires pressure monitoring in the airway.[88] Sadly, most patients with UARS remain undiagnosed and untreated.[89]

88 Barbara A. Phillips and Meir H. Kryger, 'Management of Obstructive Sleep Apnea-Hypopnea Syndrome', *Principles and Practice of Sleep Medicine*, 2011, https://doi.org/10.1016/b978-1-4160-6645-3.00110-9.

89 Gang Bao and Christian Guilleminault, 'Upper Airway Resistance Syndrome-One Decade Later', *Current Opinion in Pulmonary Medicine* 10, no. 6 (2004), https://doi.org/10.1097/01.mcp.0000143689.86819.c2.

- **Respiratory effort related to arousal (RERA):** RERAs are abrupt changes from deep to shallow sleep linked to breathing effort. They don't measure or register on the official sleep study scale, but they can be seen on breathing traces in medical sleep studies. They cause sleep fragmentation and, if occurring multiple times a night, this means sleep rest is ineffective. Negative pressures in the airway caused by obstruction can be associated with reflux. There can also be disruptions to breathing like choking and gasping. The body then wakes itself up to take a breath. Repeated episodes like this during the night can have similar consequences to OSA.[90]

- **Mouth breathing:** Mouth breathing is a habit that can develop because kids have a blocked nose, narrow nasal passages or simply because everyone around them is mouth breathing and unconscious copying occurs. It is not usually something on the parent radar, and is so common that it is both missed and considered harmless by many. Frequently, when the mouth breathing discussion is raised, parents will say their children never mouth breathe. Once they know what to look for, however, they often discover, to their surprise, that both they and their children are mouth breathing! While it might not seem important, habitual mouth breathing can lead to nasal disuse interfering with the optimum functioning of the nose and leading to congestion. Research has demonstrated that mouth breathing can lower blood oxygen levels.[91]

PARASOMNIAS

Of the sleep disorders, the most well-known are the parasomnias, which include sleep walking, talking and night terrors. Parasomnias are more frequent in children than adults because children spend more time in deep sleep. They are thought to occur in the transition from the

90 Barry Krakow, Jacoby Krakow, Victor A. Ulibarri and Natalia D. Mciver, 'Frequency and Accuracy of 'RERA' and 'RDI' Terms in the Journal of Clinical Sleep Medicine from 2006 through 2012', *Journal of Clinical Sleep Medicine*, 2014, https://doi.org/10.5664/jcsm.3432.
91 Niaki et al., 'Evaluation of Oxygen Saturation by Pulse-Oximetry in Mouth Breathing Patients'.

deep sleep of stages 3 and 4 during a micro-awakening, occurring in the first part of the night. There is a dual brain state where the body is in deep sleep but the brain is awake enough to perform other tasks. It usually happens when children are aged from four to six, and may peak between four and eight years.[92]

Parasomnias include:

- **Sleep walking and talking:** Sleep walking seems to run in families, with thirty per cent of people who sleep walk having another family member who does so, too. Meanwhile, forty per cent of children sleep walk at least once, while three to four per cent experience weekly or monthly episodes. It can be likened to doing something on automatic pilot. Kids are blissfully unaware of what is going on even if they appear to be awake, which can be distressing to parents. Other than ensuring the surrounding environment is safe, it's best to do nothing or to gently lead a child back to bed. Intervening can make the episode last longer. Sleep talking is part of the same behaviour but is naturally less risky.

- **Night terrors:** Six per cent of children experience night terrors, as distinct from nightmares. Night terrors are a highly stressful event resulting in a fast heart rate and bizarre behaviours like flailing, screaming or pushing people away. Unlike nightmares, night terrors occur in stages 3 and 4 of sleep, and on waking there is no memory or awareness of these events. There is some speculation about whether they are triggered by upper airway resistance, as they can occur more frequently in children with SDB. Sleep terrors can be very stressful and scary to parents. As children mature and deep sleep decreases, night terrors usually cease by the teenage years.

- **Nightmares:** Nightmares are not parasomnias and are different to night terrors, but they are worth mentioning here because the two are commonly mixed up. Nightmares, which peak from ages three to six,

---

92   Owens and Mindell, *Take Charge of Your Child's Sleep.*

can increase the heart rate, cause sweating and waking and trigger other sleep disruptions. They are more likely to occur in the middle of the night or early morning. Three per cent of children have recurring nightmares and, when they recur, a child may be too frightened to go to bed and too fearful to go to sleep. Both nightmares and dreams take place during REM. The most important thing is to get to the bottom of why they are occurring and develop strategies to help children manage these scary dreams. Nightmares can result from a traumatic event or underlying psychological distress. Frequent, persistent or intense nightmares may require the help of a psychiatrist or psychologist.

Parasomnias are harmless as long as physical dangers are not present, but can be frightening for parents. It can be confusing to see your child appear wide awake and wandering around the house, or there may be screaming, strange dialogue or bizarre movements, but they generally fall back to sleep very quickly once back in bed.

If a child is already prone to parasomnias, things that can make them worse include a lack of sleep, an irregular sleep schedule, late bedtimes, fever, some medications, a full bladder, a change of sleep environment, a noisy environment, stress or a sleep disorder. A medical consultation to diagnose other sleep disorders, such as SDB, may be advisable.

While parasomnias are usually benign, if you feel your child is at risk or danger or there is significant disruption to family, you may need help from a sleep specialist.

RESTLESS LEG SYNDROME

Restless leg syndrome is the overwhelming urge to move legs when lying still. It can be painful, with tingling and itching occurring at night-time. Restless leg syndrome causes the quality of sleep to be compromised because it makes it more difficult to fall asleep and leads to night-time waking. About ten per cent of adults and two per cent of children experience restless leg syndrome. Some correlation to SDB has been found.

Restless leg syndrome can be controlled with careful food choices and stretching, alongside taking medication on the advice of your medical specialist.

NARCOLEPSY

Narcolepsy involves falling asleep suddenly without warning and without control, and immediately entering REM sleep without going through the normal sequence of sleep stages. In narcolepsy, the brain is unable to control its sleep/wakefulness cycles, and 'sleep attacks' can occur anywhere, at any time. While rare, symptoms of narcolepsy can be disabling, including excess daytime sleepiness, cataplexy (sudden loss of muscle tone triggered by emotion), hypnagogic hallucinations (vivid dream experiences) and sleep paralysis. Narcolepsy has significant effects on behaviour and learning in children.

There's no cure for narcolepsy. However, medications and environmental and lifestyle changes can decrease the frequency of events.

Chronic medical and physical conditions and sleep disorders

There's a sub-group of serious sleep disorders related to chronic medical conditions and disabilities. Chronic pain, infectious disease, bacterial and viral infections, cancer, and medications used to treat medical conditions can all disrupt sleep-wake cycles or shorten sleep duration. When the body is in a healing phase, sleep duration may also be longer than usual.

Any health condition that leads to collapse of the airway, limited airway dimensions related to growth, airway blockage, poor muscle tone, cervical spine anomalies or general health problems like asthma or obesity can be problematic for sleep.[93]

Your child may be more prone to a sleep disorder like SDB because of a primary medical condition. If this is the case, it is critical to have your

---

93   David McIntosh, *Snored To Death*.

child's sleep disorder properly diagnosed and treated along with other treatments they are receiving, as sleep disorders worsen virtually every medical condition.

It is not always a medical condition that leads to airway compromise. A dental condition can also be a red flag because it signals abnormal development of the face and jaws and impacts the airway. Such non-ideal alterations are related to the growth and development of the airway, which can even begin in utero (see Chapter 5).

The following list is for your interest and is not exhaustive. Don't be too worried about the medical and dental terminology, as most of the categories can only be diagnosed or recognised by your medical or dental specialist.

Conditions that may contribute to SDB include:[94]

- **Structural abnormalities of the upper airway**: Laryngomalacia, cleft palate, choanal stenosis, choanal atresia, vocal cord palsy, retrognathia, mid-face hypoplasia, macroglossia, small nasal passages, deviated nasal septum, chest wall deformity, scoliosis, facial trauma.

- **Predisposing conditions that impact airway and skeletal development**: Tissue inflammation or nasal obstruction; adenotonsillar hypertrophy, allergy, enlarged turbinates, deviated septum, narrow nasal passages.

- **Atypical or non-ideal growth and development**: Malocclusion, retrusive chin or narrow upper jaw associated with narrowed or obstructed airway. These traits or deviations not attributable to a syndrome are called craniofacial respiratory complex (CRC) trait deficiencies, reported by Dr Kevin Boyd.[95]

94 Yvonne Pamula, Gillian M. Nixon, Elizabeth Edwards, Arthur Teng, Nicole Verginis, Margot J. Davey, Karen Waters, Sadasivam Suresh, Jacob Twiss and Andrew Tai, 'Australasian Sleep Association Clinical Practice Guidelines for Performing Sleep Studies in Children', *Sleep Medicine* 36 (2017), https://doi.org/10.1016/j.sleep.2017.03.020.

95 Sleep Disordered Breathing/Obstructive Sleep Apnea Symposium, Boston University, 2018, https://www.bu.edu/dental/ce/symposia/sleep-disordered-breathing-obstructive-sleep-apnea-symposium.

- **Neuromuscular diseases:** Muscular dystrophy or Duchenne dystrophy, myotonic dystrophy, spinal muscular atrophy. Cerebral palsy will develop some level of SDB due to the absence of normal orofacial muscle tone.

- **Craniofacial syndromes affecting the upper airway:** Pfeiffer, Treacher-Collins, Crouzon and Apert's Syndrome; Pierre Robin sequence.

- **Genetic disorders affecting respiratory control:** congenital central hypoventilation syndrome, Rett syndrome, Joubert syndrome.

- **Connective tissue diseases:** Marfans, Ehlers-Danlos syndromes.[96,97,98] Children with such genetic mutations will develop SDB related to absence of abnormal cartilage in the upper and lower jaw structures.

- **Metabolic storage disorders:** Insulin resistance, Hurler's syndrome.

Other medical and dental red flags include:

- Oligo- or hypodontia (missing teeth)
- Down syndrome
- Prader-Willi syndrome
- Koolen-de Vries syndrome
- Achondroplasia
- Leigh's Disease
- Chiari malformation[99]
- Chronic lung disease
- Epilepsy
- Face and neck burns

---

96 Christian Guilleminault, Michelle Primeau, Hsiao-Yean Chiu, Kin Min Yuen, Damien Leger, and Arnaud Metlaine, 'Sleep-Disordered Breathing in Ehlers-Danlos Syndrome', *Chest* 144, no. 5 (2013), https://doi.org/10.1378/chest.13-0174.

97 Yu-Shu Huang and Christian Guilleminault, 'Pediatric Obstructive Sleep Apnea and the Critical Role of Oral-Facial Growth: Evidences', *Frontiers in Neurology* 3 (2013), https://doi.org/10.3389/fneur.2012.00184.

98 Meir Kryger, 'Oropharyngeal Growth and Skeletal Malformations', *Principles and Practice of Sleep Medicine* (Philadelphia, PA: Elsevier, 2017), 1401–22.

99 Takuro Kitamura, Soichiro Miyazaki, Hiroshi Kadotani, Takashi Kanemura, Masako Okawa, Toshihiko Tanaka, Ichiro Komada, Taketo Hatano and Hideaki Suzuki, 'Type I Chiari Malformation Presenting Central Sleep Apnea', *Auris Nasus Larynx* 41, no. 2 (2014), https://doi.org/10.1016/j.anl.2013.07.011.

General medical issues include:

- Moderate to severe obesity
- Premature birth
- Weak immune system
- High blood pressure
- Eczema

Issues your paediatrician may diagnose include:

- Delayed milestones
- Learning problems
- Persistent bed-wetting
- Developmental delays
- Slowed growth rate
- Autism spectrum disorder (ASD)
- ADHD
- Eating issues

Your family history, along with your ethnicity, can also be red flags.[100] Children with a related family member who has OSA or another sleep disorder may have a higher chance of developing the same.

As you can see, there are many physical traits and medical causes that can contribute to sleep disorders. The peak in OSA for children, which I've noted occurs around two to four years, is primarily because of enlarged tonsils and adenoids, yet OSA can also be present from birth in premature infants and is common with birth deformities. It is also possible for kids to have imperfectly developed facial bones even if they do not have a syndrome.[101]

---

100 Anna Tessa C. Villaneuva, Peter R. Buchanan, Brendon J. Yee and Ronald R. Grunstein, 'Ethnicity and Obstructive Sleep Apnoea', *Sleep Medicine Reviews* 9, no. 6 (2005), https://doi.org/10.1016/j.smrv.2005.04.005.

101 Guilleminault and Huang, 'From Oral Facial Dysfunction to Dysmorphism and the Onset Of Pediatric OSA'.

>> One of the reasons why our kids might struggle to sleep relates to evolution and how the shape and size of the human mouth, jaw and airways have changed over time

Alongside medical and physical factors, there are other more surprising influences on our airways. Evolution, genetics and epigenetics also play a part.

Evolution and our airways

One of the reasons why our kids might struggle to sleep relates to evolution and how the shape and size of the human mouth, jaw and airways have changed over time. Why is it that as children grow, their jaws can no longer fit all thirty-two teeth by the time they are adults? Why do so many people have their wisdom teeth removed? It never used to be that way.

Anthropology, the study of human societies and cultures, informs us that our earliest ancestors had thirty-two teeth and used click languages – sounds made with whole tongue pressure and suction against the roof of the mouth. It was thought the clicks were used for survival; because the sounds they made were similar to other bush sounds, members of tribes could communicate without being detected by predators. Click language persists today in the Kalahari Bushmen. This group survived for a long period in isolation, which enabled them to preserve their language. They are being studied now by anthropologists who have had to learn the click language themselves, discovering they could only get it right if they had a broad, flat palate. In fact, the clicking technique is thought to be one of the factors to have preserved the broad, flat upper jaw structure of the Bushmen.

Kalahari Bushmen babies were exclusively breastfed on demand to six months, followed by baby-led weaning to three years. In the meantime, babies were taught to chew, chew and chew some more on tough foods. All this chewing muscle work with a highly mobile tongue are thought to be key factors in facial development, particularly in very young children, where the sutures (or joins) of the four bones of the upper jaw are very pliable and can be influenced by how the tongue and other facial muscles work around them.

Based on observation of the Kalahari Bushmen, we have learnt that our ancestors never ever had a malocclusion. Malocclusion, which literally means 'bad bite', is a problem in the way the upper and lower teeth fit together in biting or chewing. Our ancestors had straight, cavity free teeth, and never had to go to the orthodontist or dentist to get their teeth and jaws fixed. Admittedly, they didn't have orthodontists and dentists back then, but nor did they need them.[102]

This pattern changed significantly in the mid-1800s. Industrialisation and changes to agriculture introduced a softer diet with processed wheat and sugar. Not only did diet change, so did the way the muscles were used during eating and drinking. Bottle-feeding for babies came into being; it was considered progress, as it allowed mums with new babies to go to work.

This is when anthropologists noticed big changes in the way our jaws developed.[103] They started seeing smaller jaws, not enough room for crooked teeth, malocclusion and voila! Crooked teeth and cavities appeared within one generation of eating a Western diet.[104] Sleep disorders relating to the airway were born. There are no doubt other contributing factors play a role like dietary changes, allergies, sedentary lifestyles, pollution and mouth breathing, but it's interesting to note that evolution is playing a part. The speed of the changes in jaw growth cannot be accounted for by genetic modification over time, as they have happened too fast.

---

102 Sheldon et al., *Principles and Practice of Pediatric Sleep Medicine*.

103 Robert S. Corruccini, *How Anthropology Informs the Orthodontic Diagnosis of Malocclusions Causes* (Lewiston: Edwin Mellen Press, 1999).

104 Weston Price, '*Nutrition and Physical Degeneration*', April 2012, http://gutenberg.net.au/ ebooks02/0200251h.html.

Facial bone size is a major factor in determining volume of the airway, as is muscle tone in the mouth, face and throat. While we do not need to gnash our teeth to ingest food as much as our forefathers did, we certainly still need good jaw structure and well-aligned jaws and teeth for healthy airway development, bone development and muscle tone.

The way the muscles in the face and mouth are used has an impact on the development of facial structure. If muscles are floppy and weak, they are more collapsible. This is particularly relevant during the phases of sleep where deeper relaxation occur (stages 3 and 4). If the airway is already small, due to having a smaller jaw, breathing changes occur. At the same time, smaller jaws restrict the space available for the tongue, so the tongue tends to overfill the oral cavity.

Smaller jaws also lead to malocclusion, which is one of the biggest single predictors of sleep disorders, because of the way malocclusion affects the size of the airway – our breathing channel. A small, narrow upper jaw is a common abnormality that contributes to OSA.[105,106]

Because there is less space and our jaws are smaller, the airway has become crowded. When this is combined with allergies that cause swelling and congestion in the nose, the critical nasal channel component of our breathing also becomes restricted.

105 Vandana Katyal, Yvonne Pamula, Cathal N. Daynes, James Martin, Craig W. Dreyer, Declan Kennedy and Wayne J. Sampson, 'Craniofacial and Upper Airway Morphology in Pediatric Sleep-Disordered Breathing and Changes in Quality of Life with Rapid Maxillary Expansion', *American Journal of Orthodontics and Dentofacial Orthopedics* 144, no. 6 (2013), https://doi.org10.1016/j.ajodo.2013.08.015.
106 B. H. Seto, H. Gotsopoulos, M. R. Sims and P. A. Cistulli, 'Maxillary Morphology in Obstructive Sleep Apnoea Syndrome', *Eur J Orthod* 23, no. 6 (2001): 703–14.

> **>> Your experiences can modify the expression of your DNA, and these changes can be passed down through the generations**

Genetics and epigenetics

While evolution makes modern humans in general more susceptible to sleep disorders, genetics can help explain why individuals suffer. If parents have a sleep disorder it is more likely that the children will have, or get, the same one.[107,108]

However, just because a sleep disorder runs in your family, it doesn't mean your kids (or even you) are destined to suffer. In the past it was believed that genetics were immutable; you were stuck with the genes you were born into, genes that had developed by adaption to changing conditions over thousands and millions of years. However, the more recent field of epigenetics has uncovered some fascinating evidence. It shows that parts of our gene structure can be expressed differently and be modified according to environment and lifestyle factors: what we eat, how we move, how we deal with stress and how we sleep. Hardships imposed on us, such as disease, pollution and starvation, can also influence gene expression but are rarely under our control.[109] Nonetheless, for many of us, lifestyle factors are very much within our conscious control.

So, your experiences and choices in your lifetime can modify the expression of your DNA, and these changes can be passed down through the generations. One of the most interesting and controversial aspects of epigenetics is the concept of inheritance. This suggests that events in our lives can affect our children's development and health, and our grandchildren's.

107 Simon Beaulieu-Bonneau, Mélanie Leblanc, Chantal Mérette, Yves Dauvilliers and Charles M. Morin, 'Family History of Insomnia in a Population-Based Sample', *Sleep* 30, no. 12 (2007), https://doi.prg/10.1093/sleep/30.12.1739.

108 Amita Sehgal and Emmanuel Mignot, 'Genetics of Sleep and Sleep Disorders', *Cell* 146, no. 2 (2011), https://doi.org/10.1016/j.cell.2011.07.004.

109 Stephen J. Ceci, *The Nature-Nurture Debate: The Essential Readings* (Malden, Md.: Blackwell Publ., 2007).

Similarly, experiences our parents and grandparents had before we were born may also impact on our lives, another version of a 'hand-me-down'. There's a very famous well-documented case where we can clearly see the impact of famine and starvation during pregnancy in the subsequent grand-child generation.[110] While we have no control on what happened before our time, we certainly have control on the positive expression of our 'hand-me-down' genes on our children and grandchildren.

Nutrition, sleep, stress management and physical activity are all factors that can influence the 'changeable' part of our gene code. The current incidence of many sleep disorders cannot be explained by normal genetic processes and modifications over time, as the changes have taken place far too quickly. This suggests that many but not all sleep problems may be due to an epigenetic expression of our genes.

Of course, the non-changeable part of your gene code, your genetic inheritance, is not alterable with current medical techniques, but perhaps this technology is not too far away.

If the unchangeable part of your genetic structure predisposes you to certain medical conditions or growth patterns, then that is another matter. For that, we rely on good quality medical care.

For now, it is comforting to know that we can have a positive influence on our health right now, and the health of future generations, by choosing a lifestyle with optimum nutrition, exercise, sleep and physical activity, minimising exposure to pollutants. How well we do all those things will influence us and our kids today as well as the generations to come.

110   Kylie Andrews, 'Epigenetics: How Your Life Could Change the Cells of Your Grandkids', ABC News, April 21, 2017, http://www.abc.net.au/news/science/2017-04-21/what-does-epigenetics-mean-for-you-and-your-kids/8439548.

Causes of disordered sleep (as opposed to sleep disorders)

Causes of disordered sleeping can vary, and are connected to sleep environment, behaviour, habits and routines. In many cases, lifestyle is the main culprit, which means disordered sleeping can often be addressed with changes to your behaviour, environment and routine.

Irregular hours, technology overload, too many naps, not enough naps, use of medications and supplements, nutritional deficiencies, dietary habits, environmental overload, being too hot, too hungry, too stressed – all these contribute to poor sleep.

In his book *Night School*, Richard Wiseman points out that the world we live in is somewhat at fault for our sleeplessness.[111] City lights are on twenty-four hours a day, seven days a week. People, including kids, are glued to computers, phones, tablets and TVs, most of which emit blue light, which causes suppression of melatonin. Poor melatonin release doesn't only muck around with our sleep cues, but also our wider health. Melatonin lowers blood pressure, preventing heart attacks and strokes along with limiting the production of other hormones associated with cancers and diabetes, so when its release is hampered, the consequences are far-reaching.

Environment also plays a role. Take 'snoree' syndrome, for example. This is where someone's sleep is disrupted by a snorer or loud breather. Likewise, sleep disruption can be caused by someone who moves a lot. Snoring parents, grandparents or visiting relatives can wake kids up. Meanwhile, sleep monitors, which are supposed to put fearful parents' minds at rest while babies sleep, may induce avoidable sleep fragmentation for parents as they are alerted by every tiny snuffle or gurgle a baby makes. Recurring nightmares and night-time waking can be connected to what is going on in a child's day as well as to their media exposure.

---

111 Wiseman, *Night School: The Life-Changing Science of Sleep.*

The self-perpetuating cycle of disordered sleep

You should now have a much clearer picture of what good sleep should look like – and a better idea of what could be getting in the way of it for your child.

The next challenge is to figure out how to break the poor sleep cycle. Regardless of the cause of your child's disordered sleep, the trickiest piece of the puzzle is that the whole sleeplessness problem self-perpetuates. For instance, kids in pain have sleep disruption. Tired kids in pain then have trouble coping with treatments and stress. Parents then have trouble coping with the sleepless nights. And sleeplessness exacerbates every issue they are already dealing with.

>> Lifeguards, time to get out your binoculars

In order to break such an exhausting cycle, the first step is working out what kind of disordered sleep, or sleep disorder, your child is struggling with, no matter how mild. In Chapter 3, I will help you get specific and show you how to identify the red flags of a sleep problem. Lifeguards, time to get out your binoculars.

CHAPTER THREE

Recognising the red flags

'Many kids with OSA are undiagnosed.
We are only seeing the tip of the iceberg.'

– DR DAVID GOZAL[112]

I hear it all the time. Parents say, 'Little Johnny is a great sleeper.' Yet I see little Johnny sitting in front of me, lethargic, mouth open, wet face from dribbling and with black circles under his eyes. All of this tells me that Johnny is not a great sleeper – even if he is asleep for eleven hours.

Then there's little Lucy, who is constantly wired. Her parents say, 'It's just her make-up – she's a ball of energy.' Yet, looking at her sleep history, there is a firm pattern. Lucy has not had a full night's rest since she was a baby. As a toddler, she developed fears, nightmares and night terrors, and now she's seven and can barely sit still or focus or listen. She can recite her deepest fears and talks about how she wakes in the middle of the night terrified, her heart pounding, because of a monster or something she has seen on TV or heard someone talking about. She's then so terrified she cannot go back to sleep, so she crawls into bed with mum or dad or grandma (who snores), and no one gets a good sleep.

Families can become so used to a child's pattern that it becomes their new normal, even though it may be well outside the norm. But when there is not much information available to shed a light on what is normal, then everyone just soldiers on.

---

112 David Gozal, 'Pediatric Sleep Apnea: Clinical and Diagnostic Aspects', *World Sleep Society Conference* (Prague, 2017).

It's time to take a look at your children and their sleep through objective eyes so you can determine if they are sticking to the right sleep formula for their age or whether it's time to seek help.

The key is observation. This is where you get to be a lifeguard on active watch, looking for the signs signalling sleep problems. Red flags are clues about the health of your child's sleep and airways.

As we go through this chapter, you'll have the chance to examine your child from a number of angles, asking yourself such questions as:

- How does my kid behave?
- How does my kid look?
- How does my kid sound?
- How are the muscles in my kid's upper airway working?
- What medical, dental or physical condition does my kid have?

To help you look at your child's sleep objectively, I've provided charts and taken a 'workbook' approach to looking at red flags relating to your kids' sleep, night-time and daytime behaviour, airway, any medical or dental issues, environment and routine. If carers or other family members have mentioned things you have not seen, try to include their observations when you fill out the charts.

Because many things impact sleep – sleep hygiene, environment, lifestyle, stress, mental health and more – you'll be looking for red flags in a number of areas, including bedtime, night-time and daytime behaviours. If your kids, like many others, are in childcare from a young age, you can find out what's typically going on in the daytime from their carers, who will be able to tell you about sleep behaviour (naps), but also developmental factors like communication, emotional coping skills, physical ability and developing social skills.

While you are the chief lifeguard, lifeguards work best in teams, and the other lifeguards in your child's life are the people who spend a lot of time with your kids. If your child has a behaviour problem and carers, family or others suggest it may be ADHD or advise you to take your child to a paediatrician, it can be alarming. It may be your natural response to disagree with a perceived criticism. For most well-intentioned feedback about a child's behaviour, the primary driver is love and concern. Because childcare professionals are so well positioned to see many children and their interactions, try to keep this front of mind. While it can be difficult to get feedback on your children's behaviour, it can help you to pinpoint issues you may be missing. Behaviour issues are a red flag for problem sleep.

Sleep red flags

The first place to look for red flags is your child's sleep. In my clinic, I ask parents questions like: Do your children sleep well? Are your children noisy or restless sleepers? Do your children walk or talk in their sleep? Do your children struggle to get to sleep?

Many parents find it very hard to answer questions about how their children look or sound during sleep. It was never on my own radar twenty years ago when my boys were little. Most of us don't usually take a lot of notice, because we are so happy the little tackers are asleep. I find that when parents understand what to look for, they start to discover red flags. This can come as a surprise to some, as was the case with Ben.

Ben's sister, Layla, had been referred to me by her dentist because she was five years old and still sucking her thumb – a habit that would disrupt the normal growth of her upper jaw. As part of our intake process, Layla's mum filled out a questionnaire about her daughter's early development and medical and dental background.

Part of this questionnaire was looking at her sleep, at which point Layla's mum had a light bulb moment. She realised that Layla's three-year-old brother, Ben, had multiple red flags for a sleep disorder: waking several times a night, mouth breathing and snoring. His speech and language were very slow to develop – he was still only using one-word sentences – and his mum said he behaved like a little 'mad man'. While his mum was aware of her little mad man's symptoms, she was not aware of his night-time red flags, and had therefore not thought to seek help before reading the questionnaire.

I discussed these concerns with the family's GP, who then referred Ben to an ear, nose and throat specialist. As it turned out, Ben was not hearing well, had glue ear, enormous adenoids, suffered allergies and could not breathe well. The specialist decided it was an urgent matter to remove Ben's adenoids. All symptoms cleared up within three months of these being removed. His hearing returned to normal, he was breathing and sleeping well, his speech development took off and he was like a different child with a new, delightful personality. He was a healthy, energetic boy, just no longer 'wired'. However, this wouldn't have been possible if Ben and Layla's mum hadn't had the opportunity to reflect on his red flags.

In clinic, I have developed a sleep formula questionnaire for use, based on a quick question guide originally created by paediatric sleep specialist Dr Jim Papadopoulos. He used the phrase 'SSS Disturbed Rest' for new families in his sleep clinic. Dr Papadopoulos shared his method with us at a conference in Sydney in 2014,[113] and the current clinical questionnaire has evolved from there, designed to capture essential elements of the sleep formula.

This sleep questionnaire poses a range of yes/no questions about your child's sleep patterns and behaviours. Any 'yes' is an indication that more questions need to be asked. In my clinic, I look at the yes/no answers in conjunction with the child's medical and developmental history, including feedback from childcare or school. Further investigation by a medical specialist, or further night-time observations by the parents, may be recommended. Based on those observations, we may or may not recommend doing an additional questionnaire: The Sleep Disturbance Scale for Children.[114]

---

113 Jim Papdopoulos, 'Sleep Behaviour and Learning in Children', in *AACP Australian Chapter – 3rd International Symposium*, (Sydney, March 28, 2014).
114 Bruni et al., 'The Sleep Disturbance Scale for Children'.

SLEEP HISTORY SCREENING: SSS DISTURBED REST

Parent Questionnaire: Answer **yes** or **no** to each question exploring your child's sleep habits

Name: Age: (years/months)   Date:

			yes	no
S	Sleeping	can you hear your child breathing while they sleep?		
	While sleeping does your child ever...	snore?		
		appear to hold breath or stop breathing?		
		gasp or wake with a startle?		
		'work hard' to breathe		
		have their body in odd positions?		
		have their head extended back?		
		grind their teeth		
		breathe with their mouth open?		
		leave drool on the pillow?		
S	Sleepless Does your child...	have difficulty getting to sleep?		
		have difficulty staying asleep?		
		wake middle of the night and have trouble going back to sleep?		
		sleep lightly and are they easily roused		
S	Sleepy Despite adequate hours of sleep does your child...	wake slow?		
		wake groggy and moody?		
		wake with a headache?		
		experience day time sleepiness?		
		appear lethargic or hyperactive during the day?		
D	Disturbed sleep Does your child...	have nightmares?		
		have nightmares and not remember next day?		
		sleep walk or talk?		
		wet the bed?		
		toss and turn?		
R	Restless Does your child...	have fidgety legs?		
		growing pains?		
		wake in a tangle of bedclothes? Or on the wrong side of the bed?		

Q	Sleep quantity How many hours sleep does your child get, on average, in a 24-hour period including naps? Circle the number closest to the usual sleep hours your child gets	15–17	13–14	11–12	10–11	9–10
		8–9	7–8	6–7	Less than 6	
		Do you believe your child is getting enough sleep?				
Q	Sleep quality	Do you believe that your child has good Sleep Quality consistently?				

To begin looking at your child's sleep more closely, start by checking in on your child regularly every night and morning. Watch and listen. Try not to disturb them. If you can take photos or videos without disturbing your child, do so. These observations form your baselines.

After about a week, if you are seeing a consistent pattern, then fill out the questionnaire. If your child requires treatment, you can look at these again later and compare once treatment is complete. Ideally, you will notice a big change.

>> How your children sleep affects how they behave – and reciprocally, how they behave affects how well they go to sleep

If you answer any of these questions with a 'yes', and your child's sleep quantity is lower or higher than it should be for their age (see page 58), we need to dig deeper.

Behavioural red flags

How your children sleep affects how they behave – and reciprocally, how they behave affects how well they go to sleep. When sleep problems are caused by behaviour, I think of it as *disordered sleep* rather than a sleep disorder. Kids can get into habits over time that can be quite hard to break. The key questions are about who is affected and how the behaviour is affecting the sleep formula. Over the following pages, I'll share some red flags of disordered sleeping. Keep in the back of your mind that some behaviours can also signal a sleep disorder.

Night-time shenanigans

Close your eyes and imagine you are on a beautiful island for a holiday with your beautiful kids. You've had a wonderful day at the beach and, as the sun sets at 6:30pm, the kids are tired and ready for bed. They fall asleep instantly and you watch their sweet, sleeping faces for five minutes as you remember the amazing day. They sleep throughout the night, and come into your room for a snuggle after they hear you wake at 7.30am.

Doesn't that sound amazing? For many of us, it's about as far from reality as possible! But let's put a placeholder in that dream, because if you get your kids' sleep formula right, it could become a reality.

There are a number of night-time behaviours (or, as I call them, shenanigans) that signal disordered sleep. These are stalling tactics, fear of going to bed, inability to switch off or slow down enough to fall asleep, inability to stay asleep and having restless sleep.

Sometimes such behaviours can simply be a part of getting older. As children grow, their sleep needs change. As they develop language skills and test out their ability to influence those around them, this can lead to testing the limits at bedtime. I recall visiting friends many years ago who had a three-year-old girl. Little Gabby was very determined to stay up way past her bedtime, wanting to be a part of the adult conversation. When her parents put her back to bed, she protested, 'But I'm part of the family too!' It was heart-breaking, and a completely plausible reason to stay up. I take my hat off to the parents who firmly but kindly kept her in her bed and in her bedroom.

While a short phase of adjustment as a child grows and matures is one thing, long-term patterns of stalling, endless excuses, delay tactics and long sleep latency times (that is, taking a long time to go to sleep) night after night can be a behavioural, rather than developmental, issue. They can also signal a sleep disorder.

To help you assess your child's night-time behaviour, look at each trait in the table on page 93 and mark the table to note down how often you see it happening.

Daytime shenanigans

Daytime shenanigans that result from sleep disorders or not getting enough sleep can look a lot like ADHD: difficulty concentrating and focusing, aggression, impulsivity, interrupting, talking out of turn and inability to sit still. Conversely, some children can become lethargic and clumsy.

When looking at kids' behaviour, mood and frame of mind, there are lots of variations in children's personalities and they have good days and bad days, like everyone does. Sometimes I'm asked, 'Aren't most kids grumpy (or snuffly, grizzly, wired and off the planet) sometimes?' On occasions, yes, they can be, but not on a consistent basis. Kids who sleep well and wake well are happy, have energy through the day and are able to regulate their behaviour to the level expected for their age. They grow well, have great immunity and progress as expected on their developmental milestones, unless they've been diagnosed with a medical condition or other disorder.

The picture with particularly bright kids can be a bit deceiving, as bright kids that are not getting the right sleep may appear to be tracking okay when compared to others. However, they are not necessarily tracking anywhere near their best.

To determine if your children are exhibiting any daytime behavioural red flags, look at each behaviour in the table on page 94 and mark the table to note down how often this behaviour takes place.

Keep in mind that it's easy to look at your children with rose-coloured glasses. You want to see your children as perfect, which means you may be too close to see certain behaviours yourself, or you may be so used to certain behaviours that you think of them as normal. If your child spends all day at day care or school, the carers or early learning professionals may well be seeing things that you aren't. So, when filling in the chart, try to account for others' perceptions as well as your own, or even consider having your child's carers fill it out to help you gain another perspective.

How do your night-time and daytime tables look, now that you've finished filling them in?

If you have a lot of behaviours marked as 'often/usually' and 'all the time', it's time to address the underlying issues. If a child is having a bad day, that's one thing. But when a child exhibits these behaviours day in and day out and it appears to be a trait, that's when you need to think about why. If these cannot be explained easily by current life circumstances or challenges, like moving to a new house or welcoming a new baby to the family, then they're more ingrained behavioural habits.

> **>> By tuning in quickly and nipping such behaviours in the bud, you can allay unnecessary development of undesirable traits that will shape your kids' relationships and their future life**

While it's tempting to hope your kid will grow out of these traits, it's better to act early and address them. Kids who don't sleep are at risk of developing depression either now or in the future,[115] and kids who develop behavioural habits of grumpiness and aggression can hang on to those, because emotional states can become habitual and develop into the norm.[116] By tuning in quickly and nipping such behaviours in the bud, you can allay unnecessary development of undesirable traits that will shape your kids' relationships and their future life.

Environment and routine red flags

Our environments, routines and lifestyles have a big impact on how well we sleep – the same goes for our kids. Over the coming pages, you'll evaluate both for red flags.

Environment health check

When it comes to the sleeping environment, there is an optimal way to set up your child's room. This also means that there are clear red flags that can affect their sleep. Once again, look at each element in the table on page 96 and mark the table to note down how often it takes place.

115 Yasmin Anwar, 'Sleep Loss Linked to Psychiatric Disorders', UC Berkley, last modified 22 October, 2007, http://www.berkeley.edu/news/media/releases/2007/10/22_sleeploss.shtml.
116 Kheirandish-Gozal, 'Morbidity of OSA in Children'.

Health check for the bedtime routine

Like the sleeping environment, the bedtime routine also influences your child's ability to experience good sleep.

Airway red flags

Sleep disorder related to the upper airway is a common reason for kids to experience sleep problems. Airway problems lead to common characteristics that sleep-wrecked children exhibit when it comes to how they look and how they sound. Some red flags are redder than others.[117,118]

In the table on page 98, I share some of the key red flags to look for at different times of the day or night. You may need to carefully watch your child for a few days to notice anything, or even look at some photos of your child to spot things you may not be seeing day to day. I had a mother say once that she was in such a sleep fog that she stopped 'seeing'. It wasn't until she looked at a photo that she realised how utterly exhausted her child was. I have found the same thing when I look at clinic photos of kids; photos are at times more revealing than face-to-face observations.

Again, assess your child's airway using the table on page 98.

Myofunctional and dental red flags

For the table on page 100, answer the question: 'Does my child have this condition or has it been diagnosed by a dentist, orthodontist or myofunctional practitioner?' with a yes or no. When looking at a child's facial development, there may be clues that their airway is not developing in an ideal manner. They can serve as clinical markers for sleep-disordered breathing. One of the most common clues is small jaw size.[119]

---

117 Gozal, 'Pediatric Sleep Apnea: Clinical and Diagnostic Aspects'.

118 Marco Zaffanello, Giorgio Piacentini, Giuseppe Lippi, Vassilios Fanos, Emma Gasperi and Luana Nosetti, 'Obstructive Sleep-Disordered Breathing, Enuresis and Combined Disorders in Children: Chance or Related Association?' *Swiss Med Wkly*, no. w14400 (2017):147, https://smw.ch/article/doi/smw.2017.14400.

119 Guilleminault and Huang, 'From Oral Facial Dysfunction to Dysmorphism and the Onset Of Pediatric OSA'.

Medical red flags

As discussed in Chapter 2 (page 70), medical issues can also either contribute to, or be a risk factor for, a sleep disorder.[120,121,122] For this section, answer the question with a yes or a no: 'Does my child have this condition, or has it been medically diagnosed?'

How do I know how serious the problem is?

By now you should have a developing picture of whether your child is suffering from disordered sleep or a sleep disorder. However, you might be wondering how serious the problem is and whether you need to be concerned.

Like all problems, disordered sleep exists on a continuum from mild to severe. The severity may help you define your approach – if it does look severe, you might find yourself acting with urgency looking for expert assistance, whereas if it's mild you might feel like you can wait and watch for a while, put some 'fixes' in place and see if the problem resolves.

Sleep disorders carry a more immediate gravity and urgency, and any issue of this nature needs immediate action. I can't tell you how many times I have had people say to me, 'My child has OSA, but it's only mild'. The term 'mild' may be misleading. Although sixty-five per cent of children may outgrow the condition within twelve months,[123] a sleep disorder is a serious condition, and mild OSA will still have some effect. Many parents want to know what they can do and whether something can be done to mitigate the affects – and whether their child is in the sixty-five per cent. But even a diagnosis of mild OSA means that your child wakes from airway obstruction anywhere between one and five

120 Huang and Guilleminault, 'Pediatric Obstructive Sleep Apnea and the Critical Role of Oral-Facial Growth: Evidences'.

121 Bradley A. Edwards, Danny J. Eckert and Amy S. Jordan, 'Obstructive Sleep Apnoea Pathogenesis from Mild to Severe: Is It All the Same?' *Respirology* 22, no. 1 (2016), https://doi.org/10.1111/resp.12913.

122 Guilleminault et al., 'Sleep-Disordered Breathing in Ehlers-Danlos Syndrome'.

123 Scott Burgess, presentation, *AAOM Inc Symposium Day* (Coolangatta, February 17, 2018).

>> Dr Leila Kheirandish-Gozal puts it this way: 'Just imagine, someone says to your child "wake up! wake up! wake up!" five times an hour. That's what happens in sleep apnoea, every time an apnoea happens. Every night a child is not treated, is a very big problem

times every hour.[124] Dr Leila Kheirandish-Gozal puts it this way: 'Just imagine, someone says to your child "wake up! wake up! wake up!" five times an hour. That's what happens in sleep apnoea, every time an apnoea happens. Every night a child is not treated, is a very big problem.'[125]

The great news is that, as a parent who has invested time to read this book, you're someone who takes the role as 'sleep lifeguard' earnestly and you're ready and willing to take action. What's more, your action can be targeted and informed, thanks to your careful observation of your child and your growing familiarity with their sleep red flags. In the next chapter, I'll share some things you can do to start improving your child's sleep.

---

124 Eleonora Dehlink and Hui-Leng Ta, 'Update on paediatric obstructive sleep apnoea', *The Journal of Thoracic Disease* 8, no. 2 (2016).

125 Kheirandish-Gozal, 'Morbidity of OSA in Children'.

NIGHT-TIME SHENANIGANS

TRAITS at night		My child is like this:				
		never	rarely	occasionally	often	always
In the lead-up to bed time – my child	gets a second wind: is wound up or wired					
	is unable to follow easy instructions					
	becomes teary or grumpy					
	refuses to get ready for bed					
	falls asleep in places other than bed					
Going to bed and to sleep – my child	refuses to go to bed					
	becomes agitated					
	uses delay tactics and excuses					
	is unable to go to sleep without being held or having someone in the room					
	is unable to wind down					
	is afraid to go to sleep					
	takes more than 10-15 minutes to go to sleep					
	has difficulty falling to sleep					
Once asleep – my child	wakes and calls out at night					
	wakes and gets into someone else's bed during the night ('musical beds')					
	wakes and is afraid					
	gets into strange body positions					
	wakes numerous times					
	sleeps lightly/easily roused					
	wakes and is unable to go back to sleep					
	wakes or talks during sleep					
	has nightmares					

DAYTIME SHENANIGANS

TRAITS during the day – my child		My child is like this:					
		never	others see it	rarely	occasionally	often	always
Emotional	is grumpy						
	is a worrier						
	is irritable						
	is scared/fearful						
	is sad						
	is short tempered						
	is sensitive						
	is unable to see 'reason'						
	has sudden mood swings						
	has emotional outbursts						
Social	is uncooperative						
	is prone to fights						
	appears not to listen						
	is clingy						
	is argumentative						
	interjects/interrupts a lot						
	does not like the word 'no'						
	has difficulty making or keeping friends						
	is oppositional or defiant						
Learning	is easily distracted						
	is unable to focus, concentrate or pay attention						
	is 'spaced out', a dreamer						
	does not communicate as well as other kids the same age						
	is 'behind other kids of the same age						
	is not doing as expected for ability level						
	is challenged by problem solving						
	can't follow instructions						

DAYTIME SHENANIGANS

TRAITS during the day – my child		My child is like this:					
		never	others see it	rarely	occasionally	often	always
Behaviour	is whingey and whiney						
	is unmotivated						
	is agitated						
	is easily frustrated if unable to do something						
	is wired						
	is disruptive						
	can be aggressive or a bully						
	is forgetful						
	behaves like a child with ADHD						
	appears not to listen or hear						
	is unable to regulate undesirable behaviour						
Physical	avoids activities like swimming/running						
	falls asleep at inopportune times						
	can't sit still						
	constantly on the move						
	fidgets excessively						
	is lethargic						
	is sleepy						
	has a lot of energy						

MY CHILD'S SLEEP ENVIRONMENT

ENVIRONMENTAL FACTORS My child or my child's...	The environment is like this:				
	never	rarely	occasionally	often	always
room is noisy at sleep time					
sleeps with a light on					
room is hard to keep cool or warm (season dependent)					
goes to bed upset					
sleeps with a pet					
says they get cold during the night					
says the bed covers are too hot					
kicks off the bed covers					
says they can't get warm					
goes to bed in a 'hyper emotional' house					
room has no blinds to keep summer light, street light or early morning light out of the room					
complains her/his pyjamas are uncomfortable					
says he/she feels scared going to bed					
has screen time within an hour of their bedtime					
has a TV or screen in the bedroom					
seems affected by our current family challenges					
alert at bedtime, there's a lot going on in the house					
appears upset by events going on in the family at the moment					
shares their room when we have visitors					
shares a room with a restless or noisy sleeper					

MY CHILD'S SLEEP ROUTINE

My child...	The routine is like this:				
	never	rarely	occasionally	often	always
goes to bed at a different time every night					
chooses their own bedtime					
has a snack right before bed					
drinks barely any or no water during the day					
has an unpredictable routine in the leadup to bedtime					
has no 'wind down' activities before sleep, e.g. bedtime story, bath, meditation					
is not sure how to get ready for bed by him/herself					
refuses to go to bed when asked					
resists going to bed					
is revved up and energised at bedtime					
demands a drink before bed or during the night					
insists on 'lights on' at bedtime and during the night					
stalls or uses delay tactics at bedtime					
falls asleep in places other than their own bed					
needs lots of help and coaxing getting ready for bed					
calls out asking for things once in bed before sleep					
takes more than 15 minutes every night to fall asleep					
takes more than 30 minutes every night to fall asleep					
wakes in the middle of the night and comes into parent's or sibling's bed					
wakes in the middle of the night and cannot go back to sleep without a parent to help					
has to be woken in the morning					
is grumpy and slow to wake in the morning					

AIRWAY RED FLAGS						
TRAITS		My child is like this:				
		never	rarely	occasionally	often	always
Once asleep: what do you **hear**? – my child	appears to hold breath or stop breathing					
	gasps for air					
	snores					
	wakes with a startle or gasp					
	makes choking sounds					
	has short, fast breathing					
	has to be upright to sleep					
	has audible or loud breathing					
	grinds their teeth					
Once asleep: what do you **see**? – my child	works hard to breathe (see chest or tummy straining)					
	has their body in odd positions					
	has their head extended back					
	appears to be 'breath-holding'					
	sweats					
	wakes sitting up in bed					
	tosses and turns or has fidgety legs					
	breathes with an open mouth					
	drools on the pillow					
Once asleep: what **happens**? – my child	has nightmares					
	sleeps lightly/easily roused					
	has parasomnias (walks or talks in sleep)					
	wets the bed					
	sleeps in unusual positions (e.g. snail)					
	has strings of saliva on their shoulder or pillow					

AIRWAY RED FLAGS						
TRAITS		**My child is like this:**				
		never	rarely	occasionally	often	always
On waking: what **happens?** – my child	has morning headaches					
	wakes slowly					
	is moody					
	looks tired					
	has to be woken					
	wakes in a tangle of bed clothes					
	is groggy					
	is tired in the day, despite long sleep hours					
	avoids physical activities					
	has poor morning appetite					

MYO FUNCTIONAL & DENTAL RED FLAGS

TRAITS	How does your child look? How does your child sound? How do your child's muscles work?	My child is like this:		
		Yes	No	I don't know
How the face mouth and throat look – my child has	puffy eyes			
	dark circles			
	dry lips			
	short upper lip that barely moves			
	a lower lip that dominates or sits out from the upper lip			
	tongue sits low and forward or is out of the mouth			
	tongue is always visible			
	tendency to drool, has a wet mouth or lips or rash around the mouth or wet shirt			
	If you are not sure about the following, have a professional examination. Ask your dentist, orthodontist or orofacial myofunctional practitioner. **Examination found:**			
	Face: long, narrow face shape			
	lower jaw looks 'set back' or small			
	middle face bones or cheeks are flat/under-developed			
	weak or droopy facial muscles			
	small face, small mouth			
	lower jaw growing down and back rather than forward			
	found facial 'thirds' (horizontal, not in harmony)			
	found facial 'fifths' (top to bottom not in harmony)			
	Mouth: inside the mouth looks crowded and 'full of tongue'			
	tongue tie or other tethered oral tissues (TOTs)			
	a cross-bite			
	an open bite			
	an over jet			
	an overbite			
	an upper jaw that is high arched and narrow			
	scalloped or geographic tongue			
	'missing' teeth (agenesis)			
	late teeth eruption			
	unexplained tooth decay			
	Throat: elongated uvula			
	examination found enlarged tonsils (not necessarily tonsillitis)			
	found enlarged adenoids (X Ray)			
	narrow faucial arches			
	'low hanging' velopharynx			
	distance from back of tongue to pharynx appears restricted			

MYO FUNCTIONAL & DENTAL RED FLAGS

TRAITS	How does your child look? How does your child sound? How do your child's muscles work?		My child is like this:		
			Yes	No	I don't know
How the face mouth and throat **sound** – my child	Speech:	sounds 't', 'd', 'n', 'l', 's' and 'z' are made with the tongue too far forward			
		speech distortions because of tongue position; 'sh', 'ch', 'j', 'zh', 'r'			
		unexplained speech delays			
	Resonance:	blocked 'stuffy' nose sound			
		sounds like air is escaping through the nose during speech			
	Voice:	rough deep or hoarse voice			
	has a coughing and throat clearing habit				
	has audible breathing				
	becomes breathless with activity				
How the muscles of the face mouth and throat **work** – my child or – my child's	breathes through their mouth				
	chews their food fast				
	barely chews				
	chews with an open mouth				
	has food left over in the mouth after swallowing				
	chews noisily				
	avoids eating chewy/crunchy food				
	eats mostly soft texture food				
	swallows noisily				
	makes a facial grimace or tightens their lip/chin muscles while swallowing				
	has a tongue thrust swallow				
	tongue is visible while talking/eating				
	has their tongue out a lot while playing or concentrating				
	has a forward head posture				
	has a slumped posture				
	dribbles and drools				
	drinks regularly from a spouted/sippy cup				
	drinks regularly from any spout or baby bottle				
	sucks their thumb/finger/dummy or other objects				

MEDICAL RED FLAGS

These are things your GP or medical specialist may have diagnosed or you may consult with them about your child. Does my child have...	My child is like this:			
	Yes	If yes, describe	No	I don't know
Structural abnormality of the upper airway with underlying medical diagnosis				
Predisposing conditions including: any airway tissue inflammation				
Atypical or non-ideal airway growth and development (not syndrome) (see myofunctional and dental red flags)				
Cranio-facial syndrome				
Neuromuscular disease				
Genetic disorder				
Connective tissue disease				
Metabolic storage disorder				
Other medical or dental red flags				
Other upper airway issues				
Nasal obstruction, frequently blocked nose				
Middle ear fluid (effusion)				
Coughing at night				
Reflux or history of reflux				
Stuffy, nasal voice				
Hoarse or deep voice				
Sinus				
Habitual cough/throat clearing				
Other medical				
Weak immune system, always sick, seems to catch everything, 'out of sorts'				
High blood pressure				
Eczema				
Obesity				
Your paediatrician diagnosed				
Delayed milestones				
Difficulty with pre-literacy and numeracy				
Difficulty with literacy and numeracy				
Bedwetting continues, even though day training is successful				
General developmental delays				
Height and weight not as expected for age				
Autism spectrum				
ADHD or other behavioural issues				
Eating difficulties/restricted diet/sensory issues/ food intolerances				
Family history				
Ethnicity (Asian or Afro-American)				

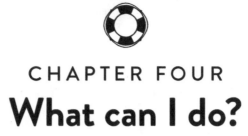

CHAPTER FOUR

What can I do?

When looking for solutions for sleep problems, it's tempting to turn straight to an expert. But there is much you may be able to do before seeking expert help. As a parent, you are in the prime seat to make little tweaks or big changes. You are there when your child is born and for their first cry and first smile. You are there when they wake and go to bed, get sick or have a meltdown, take their first steps, speak their first words and eat their first solid foods. You are there when they have a tantrum in the supermarket or crawl into your bed at some ungodly hour of the night. You are the central figure in your child's life and they in yours: you want the very best start in life for them and to give them the best chance of reaching their full potential. No one will prioritise your child's future as much as you.

This puts you in the perfect position to be the lifeguard of your child's sleep.

How can you do it?

The first step is developing sleep literacy, which you have been doing by reading this book. You now understand what good sleep looks like, the negative consequences of bad sleep and the particular red flags that are an issue for your child. The next step is looking at things you can do to improve sleep for your child. Just as a beach lifeguard creates a safe section of the beach for people to swim, you can create a safe environment at home – both the physical and emotional – in order to encourage great sleep. And just as a beach lifeguard teaches the beach-safe behaviours to swimmers, you as sleep lifeguard can establish a healthy set of routines so kids can sleep well.

In this chapter, we'll take a look at some of the clearest, most effective ways you can ensure great sleep for your child. All of these techniques are within your own control as a parent – and each of them can reap profound benefits when applied consistently within the home.

Physical environment

There are many things you can do to set up your child for sleep success, but one of the most important is making sure that conditions both inside and outside the bedroom are conducive to sleep. Noises, light, temperature and even smells can disrupt your child's ability to go to sleep or stay asleep. Being hungry, thirsty, or in pain can all lead to sleep disruption.

>> Turning the bedroom into a sleep sanctuary and following a consistent 'go to bed' routine makes a big difference in just two to four weeks

Creating a great sleep environment helps to set positive associations with sleep, which, when used regularly, become triggers for sleep. In other words, by creating a range of environmental signals, you can train the body and mind to know instinctively that it is time to sleep.

When a good sleep environment is combined with a good sleep routine, you will be well on your way to mastering the good sleep formula. Turning the bedroom into a sleep sanctuary and following a consistent 'go to bed' routine makes a big difference in just two to four weeks.

Here are some ways you can create a sleep sanctuary for your kids:

- **Light:** Light in your environment can assist or disrupt sleep cycles. If your internal clock does not register light cues, you may experience an irregular or drifting circadian rhythm. Your circadian rhythm is your own personal internal sleep clock that determines the timing and rhythm of your tiredness and sleep cycles over a twenty-four-hour period. Problems can lead to either delayed or advanced sleep phase disorders. An example of this is jetlag, which puts your body on a delayed or advanced sleep phase pattern, out of sync with your current time zone. The wrong kind of light, such as that emitted by electronic screens, will switch off melatonin, delaying and interfering with sleep onset. Darkness signals the release of melatonin. To address this, ensure you and your kids are not exposed to any bright lights or screens for at least an hour before bedtime. If you are able to dim the lights throughout the house, start turning them down an hour before bed. Ideally, your child's bedroom will be dark or have very soft lighting. This starts melatonin activation and signals the brain that sleep time is coming. If your kid needs a nightlight, a small one in a dim rosy colour will be best. Phase light out when you can. One mum told me she has a small soft lamp on a timer, which fades slowly to complete darkness over ten minutes. Complete dark is best. Some houses need blinds or curtains that completely block either street light or extended seasonal evening light.

- **Noise:** Harsh or stimulating sounds can keep us awake or rouse us from sleep. These include sounds from a TV, iPad or phone, family members talking loudly (or fighting), household noises like washing dishes, noisy neighbours, barking dogs, cars, wind and storms or music. Soft sounds, however, can help ease children into sleep. Consider using quiet, gentle classical music, white noise machines or ambient nature noises like waves and running water to mask household noise. Avoid relaxation tracks with irregular sounds like gongs or chimes. Soft sounds can mask other household and neighbourhood noise and set the scene for restful sleep.

- **Temperature:** The ideal sleep temperature is 18°C (64.4°F). Higher or cooler temperatures can lead to sleep deprivation, stress and parasomnias. It can be a delicate balance, finding the correct weight of sleep wear (pyjamas) and the correct bedding such that your child's body can maintain an even temperature through the night so they don't get too hot (and kick off the bedding) or too cold overnight. If possible, an even room temperature through the night and natural lightweight fibres for pyjamas and bedding (doonas and blankets) are ideal. In a warm climate with no temperature control, minimal bedclothes and a light fan may be the perfect combination for sleep. In a cold climate where there is no heating at night, warm natural fibre bedding that can insulate the body well will keep a child warm for the night.

- **Safety:** Children who experience regular nightmares can find bedtime very stressful. You can help them feel safe in their rooms by doing a safety check on the windows and doors, or even 'sweeping the room' with an 'invisible light sabre' to keep imaginary monsters away. Happy photos next to the bed (warm, smiling photos of loved ones or pictures of great holidays) can help, as can a soft cuddly toy. Kids need to feel safe and secure physically and emotionally. The 'emotional charge' in the household at bedtime may also contribute to how safe your child feels when it's time to say good night. Whether or not your child has had exposure to alarming news or scary events and characters in a movie during the day may also influence their sense of safety.

- **Smells:** Choose scents associated with love and safety, or essential oils that soothe and relax, like lavender or rose. Using the same smell regularly can help develop an association between smell and sleep, making it easier for your children to drift off.

- **Clutter:** Bedrooms should be a space for sleep, but many children's bedrooms are also play areas, cluttered with toys, games, electronics and other stimulating items. If you can, create a play area for all of these items outside the bedroom. If this isn't possible, packing everything up for sleep can be part of the bedtime routine. Keep any electronic screens outside the bedroom.

- **Comfort:** Choosing pyjamas and blankets with soft, hypoallergenic material can help soothe kids. Look for pyjamas with no seams for sensitive kids, or pyjamas and blankets with added scent for kids who respond to soft scents. If pyjamas have favourite characters on them, this can even give the pyjamas special meaning. For example, a superhero print could become special protective pyjamas with a 'built-in monster deterring force field' if your child is afraid of monsters.

>> A calm, loving home where a child feels safe and loved is the best environment for sleep, while an emotionally charged, chaotic or volatile household can make it hard for them to truly relax

Emotional environment

The emotional environment of your home can also affect how well (or poorly) everyone sleeps. A calm, loving home where a child feels safe and loved is the best environment for sleep, while an emotionally charged, chaotic or volatile household can make it hard for them to truly relax. It will be difficult for a child in such an environment to wind down from being excited or scared.

Insomnia commonly occurs with stressful or changing life events, ranging from more benign things like changing the clocks for daylight savings, moving to a new house or going on holidays, to bigger life events like a new baby or a terminally ill grandparent, to catastrophic events like disasters: floods, earthquake, bush fires, war. Benign life changes can be adapted to relatively easily, while significant catastrophic events can create deep anxiety, trauma and strong negative associations around sleep.

Anxiety can interfere with a child getting to sleep, staying asleep and having peaceful dreams. Kids may also find it hard to be alone. Developing strategies to cope with anxiety and building positive sleep associations are key for minimising sleep struggles. Kids who are exposed to catastrophic events may benefit from professional counselling and support, and many may require the support over an extended period of time – months rather than weeks.

It is also important to work out whether your child's anxiety is a temporary phase of adjusting to life events, or whether there is more generalised anxiety that features throughout your child's day and activities on a regular basis. The extent of the anxiety will determine the length and type of intervention required. In some cases, a good paediatric psychologist (ideally one who is specialised in sleep) may be needed.[126]

There is plenty you can do to help soothe your children into sleep:

- **Provide a favourite stuffed animal or security blanket:** Many children take to a transitional object, such as a bear or special blanket, in early childhood. This is not something to worry about and indeed can be encouraged, because such objects help a child transition from dependence to independence. These beloved objects provide a way for children to be soothed and comforted in the face of the separation anxiety that can occur at night-time. Attachment to toys and special objects varies from child to child and can't be forced, so it's best to follow your child's lead here.

- **Relax with a bedtime story before sleep:** Reading stories at night can provide a great sense of security and connection between child and parent.[127] If a child has fears or if they are facing a difficulty of some kind, you can read a story like *Orion and the Dark* by Emma Yarlett, or you could get creative and construct your own story, individualised for your child, that will interact with their dreams and integrate resilience and coping into their thinking. One of my clinic kids surmounted a scared phase because his soft toy puppy, 'Gruffy', had the power to make all scary things become super tiny just by saying the sentence, 'You are smaller and smaller and smaller and now you are invisible. Great, you are gone – now don't come back.' Helping kids develop phrases that give them a sense of control is very

126 Owens and Mindell, *Take Charge of Your Child's Sleep*, 132–33.
127 Zuania Ramos, 'Storytelling Can Help Your Children Sleep Better and Strengthen Your Family', Huffington Post, last modified August 27, 2013, http://www.huffingtonpost.com.au/entry/3817198.

affirming. Stories that promote safe feelings, create the mood for sleep and lay daytime challenges and bad moods to bed (literally) can be gold. Bedtime stories can also contain life's lessons – *Aesop's Fables* is one example. Our dreams are suggestible states, so bedtime reading is an ideal way to share stories and ideas we want our children to learn from a young age, which will help their dreams do the important ongoing work of building emotional literacy and resilience. You will find a list of suggested stories for you in Appendix B.

- **Practise relaxation techniques with your child:** Progressive relaxation, where body parts are squeezed tight then released, can help kids to let go of any physical tensions in their bodies. You simply need to talk your child through squeezing and releasing each body part: 'Squeeze your toes really tight and count to five … keep squeezing hard, harder, harder, harder, now release … aaaah, that feels good, now it feels all soft and heavy.' Repeat for all major body parts – legs, arms, face, whole body. Using words to describe the feeling helps to promote body relaxation. For a slightly different approach, check out a book called *Sleepy Little Yoga* by Martina Selway. This book contains calming poses that won't rev up your kids.

- **Do meditation together:** Meditation is a fabulous activity to include as part of the night-time routine for kids who take longer to settle. You can be inventive and create guided imagery meditations that will take your child on a journey of wonder: cloud travel or undersea secret treasure hunts, fairy gardens that wave magic sleep dust, caves where you can find your name on a giant diamond or fireflies that write your name in the night sky. Use anything that you think might capture you child's imagination. Meditation before sleep can create a special bond between parents and children. A resource I have found very useful is the Insight-timer app, which has some lovely children's 'go to sleep' meditations and stories. One of my favourites is the 'Firefly Meditation for Peaceful Sleep' by Liesl Van der Hoven.[128] During meditation, you can also teach your children a calming breathing technique.[129]

- **Clear out the monsters:** If your child is afraid of monsters or scary things, you can help to clear them out with a 'clearing ritual'. Again, we are getting creative – different things work for different children. Try using 'magic' sprays for bedroom clearance when littlies are too scared to go to sleep because of monsters. You might have blue spray for big monsters, yellow spray for smelly monsters and green spray for all other monsters! You can make these up in little bottles with water and food colouring. One spray makes them go away, and for good measure two sprays makes their pants fall down. Making kids laugh can dispel fear and anxiety. You can also have a range of 'invisible tools'. I've used some of the following successfully with one of my own kids: magic dust, spells, and an invisible sledgehammer to sweep the room, under the bed and the window where monsters could 'sneak in'. This does require a little inventiveness on your part to match the right tool for your child without overdoing it. Whatever you choose, it needs to be believable and reassuring for your particular little person.

- **Provide reassurance:** Kids' most common night-time fears are darkness, monsters, unexplained noises and intruders. It's important to reassure your child that they are safe, but if you overdo the reassurance they may think you also think a monster is real, which can make them more scared. It's a fine line. Dealing with this is somewhat dependant on their emotional and developmental maturity, the way you respond and the words you use: 'To be able to deal with fears effectively, your children need to have a well-developed sense of time ("when will I see mummy and daddy again?"), be able to

---

128 See https://insighttimer.com/FairyCaravan/guided-meditations/firefly-meditation-for-peaceful-sleep.

129 A great resource for teaching kids breathing is accessible on the Buteyko Method for Children and Teenagers website, which you can find at http://buteykoclinic.com/buteykochildren.

control emotional impulses, reason consciously and trust rational conclusions over imagination.'[130] It's also important to acknowledge your child's emotions without escalating or dismissing, and recognise real fear from a stalling tactic. You should reassure and reaffirm children that they live in a secure and safe house. At the same time, you want to build their coping skills, so in the daytime, teach them how to manage fears: one good method is to talk it through, draw the scary thing, then throw the scary thing in the bin. This can help kids resolve their fear and feel more in control. If fears persist, part of the bedtime routine can be to do a 'clearing', using words that help scary thoughts and monsters go away for good. 'This is not your house, now off you go.' However, persistent fears may require professional help.

- **Analyse the cause and address it directly:** If your child has issues that trigger poor sleep onset, helping them get to sleep can be as simple as removing the triggers and associations while you develop a new habit. It may take some thought and planning to do daytime activities that directly address the issue. First, consider what is creating daily stress: is it an over-packed schedule, an unfamiliar routine or too much screen time stimulation? It is important to avoid frightening television, stories, and imagery, especially before bedtime but also during the day. If your kid suffers from an irrational fear, talk to them about the difference between fantasy and reality and show them deep inside the wardrobe and under the bed to demonstrate, gently and patiently, that there's no beast in there. Teach coping skills through role playing.

Kids whose anxieties override these strategies may need to see a psychologist or suitable qualified health professional who can assist with anxiety management. We'll look more at this in Chapter 6.

---

130 Gwen Dewar, 'Night-Time Fears in Children: A Guide for the Science-Minded', *Parenting Science*, accessed January 1, 2018, https://www.parentingscience.com/nighttime-fears.html.

GOING DEEPER: DREAMS AND NIGHTMARES

We all dream, whether we remember our dreams or not. Our dreams are usually filled with people we are familiar with. Unfortunately, negative emotions feature frequently and family conflict and scary or traumatic events can trigger nightmares, so if you cannot work out what may be triggering your child's scary dreams, it's worth speaking to carers or others who spend time with your child to get to the bottom of the issues. The longer nightmares persist, the more likely it is that your child will start to get scared of going to bed, so it's best to address them as soon as possible.

Nightmares are scary, but it doesn't mean they are all bad. In fact, nightmares or scary dreams are the brain's way of learning to deal with difficult emotions. That being said, they remain very unsettling to littlies. Most kids have them, with twenty-four per cent of children aged two to five having chronic nightmares that last more than three months.[131]

The most important thing is to differentiate between persistent nightmares that reflect underlying anxiety and temporary nightmares triggered by daytime events. Young children are usually afraid of imaginary things that can't actually hurt them, such as being alone, the dark, imaginary creatures, monsters and thunder.[132] Kids also worry about real things that can actually hurt them like bodily injury, blood and needles. These real things can feature in dreams and nightmares.

Many kids are sensitive to media. For instance, during the bushfires in Australia there was a spike in referrals to sleep specialists due to night-

131 Owens and Mindell, *Take Charge of Your Child's Sleep*.
132 Ibid.

mares and anxiety. One little person, five-year old Billie, used to wake covered in sweat from head to toe and had frequent daytime tantrums. It was all fixed by eliminating any TV an hour before bed and replacing it with reading or another quiet activity.

Fortunately, the brain can be trained to think about and react to a nightmare differently. So once your child has an opportunity to talk about a bad dream, you can help them think about it in a new way. I suggest using the following tactics:

- **Bring humour to the situation:** Use clearing sprays that make a monster's pants fall down, while 'twinkle dust' makes monsters sneeze, giggle, run away or wet their pants.

- **Rewrite a bad dream:** Littlies can use craft and drawing and play acting to work out what happened in the dream and how it can happen differently. Go over it again and again until it becomes the new story.

- **Create a protector:** 'Fireflies in a jar' can protect littlies from the bad dreams. You can make your own http://www.beebee.info/doityourself/diy-fireflies-in-a-jar-night-lamp.

- **Meditation and visualisation:** Meditation and stories before bed can also influence dreams. (See earlier in the chapter.)

- **Introduce a third-party helper:** I'll get to this at the end of the chapter.

And of course, a consistent bedtime routine can help children feel calm, cherished and secure, which goes a long way to reducing nightmares caused by anxiety.

Routine

Everything you do in the daytime and leading up to bedtime can influence the body's ability to tune into signals that tell the brain it's time to sleep. What do your kids eat throughout the day? What do or don't they eat? How much exercise do they get? How much exposure to daylight do they have? Have your kids experienced any upsetting events or events that revved them up? Are they frightened when they can't sleep? Did a parent get upset and yell at them? Were they in trouble at school? Bullied? Hurt?

Consistent, healthy routines throughout the day and before bed are very comforting. They are key to establishing good sleep behaviour and work well to help kids adjust to changes that occur with daylight savings, visitors in the house or parents' comings and goings for work and travel. Consistent routines can help you all become 'super sleepers', where everyone gets a good night's sleep.

While establishing a routine can feel like a lot of work, especially if you and your kids are sleep deprived, it is worth putting the time and energy into getting it right as early as possible in a child's life. But if you've lived a routine-free life up until this point, it's never too late to start! (If you have a baby, look at Appendix A.)

Where to start?

Before we get into specific daytime and bedtime routines, there are some general principles that will help you and your family establish and maintain new routines.

First, don't try to change everything at once – this can cause more stress for you and your kids. Aim to adjust nap and go-to-sleep times incrementally, which may take a bit of planning and thought as kids get closer to school age. Similarly, adjustment to daylight savings may take a little time, but planning changes to your kids' environment and routine over a period of four to seven days makes the adjustment easier for everyone (particularly if they were already in a good routine). Gradual changes make the transition easier for everyone and will help avoid over-tiredness.

Second, discussions about bedtime are non-negotiable. There can be choices around pre-bed activities, but bedtime itself and the routine should remain the same. Both parents need to be on board with the system – otherwise it will be more likely that one of you will break the routine. Of course, we don't want routines to be so rigid that a child is unable to cope with change. So, the weekend may be the time when things are done *a little* differently. But at night, the aim should be for a consistent routine no matter who is helping out with bedtime. Keep in mind that managing siblings of different ages requires setting fair rules and expectations for older children who may need time with their parents after littlies have gone to bed. One idea is to involve older siblings in putting littlies to bed, which can be a special bonding experience.

Third, give it some time. Set a time to start your new routine when there isn't likely to be any disruption for at least two weeks. Don't start it if someone is sick, or there is family challenge or if a relative will be visiting. Then dedicate a good month to following your new routine to the letter – no interruptions, no changes, no excuses. In most cases, you will see improvements in two to four weeks.

Finally, if the routine is consistent for over two weeks and your kids are still not towing the line, you may need to look further into why. It might turn out that a wired kid needs a little more time and more tangible rewards for changing their behaviour. Or if stalling behaviour is causing family conflict and tension, a specialist psychologist may be able to help unravel the tension and get to the bottom of the resistance. Remember, there is always the possibility that kids are delaying bed because sleep has become unpleasant due to a sleep disorder rather than a behavioural issue, so keep an eye out for those red flags.

Once the routine is set, it will start to work by association. That is, if you stick to the routine, the routine itself will trigger sleep. Some routines become even shorter, because the brain learns to short-circuit falling to sleep and fall asleep faster, as it recognises different parts of the routine. If you are travelling and your kids struggle with sleeping in unfamiliar surrounds and beds, maintaining the same routine as you do at home can make things much easier.

Bedtime routine tips

Putting tired, cranky littlies to bed tests most parents' skills and patience. What should be a time of calm can turn into a marathon of negotiations and excuses – 'I'm not tired', 'I'm thirsty', 'I need to go to the toilet', 'I'm part of the family too', and more. Hence Adam Mansbach's book was born.[133]

Your child's bedtime routine should start at the same time every evening. To work out the best regular bedtime for your child, you'll need to 'reverse engineer' your day. Work out the time your kids need to get up in the morning (or the time they always get up), count back the ideal number of hours of sleep for their age, and that will give you the time they need to be asleep. Then count back another half an hour for the routine and fifteen minutes for them to get to sleep, and you will have a starting time for their bedtime routine every night.

For example, if you have a four-year-old child, their recommended sleep time is around twelve hours. If they take a one-hour nap during the day, that brings the amount of evening sleep they need down to eleven hours. If they wake up at 6:30am, their bedtime routine would therefore need to start at 6:45pm.

- 6:45pm: Start bedtime routine.
- 7:15pm: Tuck in to bed.
- 7:15–7:30pm: Time to fall asleep.
- 7:30pm–6:30am: Eleven hours of sleep.

---

133 Mansbach and Cortés, *Go the F**k to Sleep.*

Here are some activities you can include:

- **Bath:** A warm bath at least half an hour before bed helps the body fall asleep. Our body temperature cools down after a bath, and this drop in temperature is a trigger for the body to go to sleep. Meanwhile, brushing teeth and going to the toilet are essential activities that ought to be added to the routine after the bath.

- **A snack:** Snacks like oatmeal, a banana or milk are on the recommended list for kids who need a snack an hour before bed. Avoid caffeinated snacks such as chocolate, tea or cola at least four hours before bedtime.

- **Reading/story time:** Reading is a good, quiet activity kids and adults can do before bed. However, it's ideally done *out* of bed so that reading in bed is not associated with going to sleep. Because you are developing associations that can be used middle of night if they wake, it may not be feasible to read a story to them each time they wake and need to go back to sleep. If reading in bed is your preference, however, finish the story just before they fall asleep. You can say, 'I see you are ready for sleep now. Night-night and sweet dreams.'

- **Other 'wind-down' activities:** Yoga for little people can stretch and unwind muscles and slow down busy brains

- **List for tomorrow:** Making lists for the next day can help quell anxiety. They are also useful for little 'chatterboxes' who start talking as soon as they get into bed. Have a notepad and write it down before getting into bed: 'Will talk about the dinosaur picnic with Lily in the morning.'

- **Movement:** Rocking facilitates deep sleep. You can have a cuddle on a rocking chair, or babies can rock on a tummy-time pod.

- **Touch:** Cuddles, gentle patting and massage can help soothe kids before bed and allow for special bonding time.

- **Music and meditation:** You and your child could listen to a guided meditation or some soft music before going to bed.

- **Saying goodnight:** If you have a larger family with older siblings or extended family in the home, littlies can kiss everyone good night before going to bed. They can also say goodnight to their toys and games as part of an evening clean up.

- **Banish the monsters:** If your child is going through a scared phase, you can banish the monsters together as part of your routine.

Bedtime should be a special, enjoyable time that kids look forward to without getting too hyped up.

Once a bedtime routine is set, the time required for the routine decreases as the brain adapts and associations trigger the process of 'falling to sleep'. Once a routine is well established, it becomes possible to change a routine temporarily and then return to it. If you are travelling and it is hard to stick to the exact routine, make sure you return to it as soon as you are home. While you are away, stick to the routine as much as possible as it can help when sleeping in unfamiliar surrounds and beds.

GOING DEEPER: WHEN HELPING YOUR CHILD GET TO SLEEP BECOMES A PROBLEM

Many parents feel torn between wanting a warm, cuddly and loving bedtime and wanting their child to learn to fall asleep on their own. Research indicates that forty-three per cent of parents stay with their preschool child and twenty-three per cent stay with their school-aged child until they drift off to sleep. The chances are that if you do this, they'll need you again if they wake middle of the night.[134]

If lying with your child to help them go to sleep is what you want to do, it is a personal choice. Many parents start this and then find that it becomes very difficult to sustain. It can become increasingly long with more and more demands from the children, eroding parents' own wind-down time at the end of the day.

Love can be shown in many ways, and your most powerful tool at bedtime is a warm, loving voice and reassuring manner. If you have been lying down with your child for a long time, you have become their 'cuddly'. Many kids have a teddy or cuddly toy of some kind, but if you have become their teddy bear you're in a bit of a bind, as this habit is difficult to sustain and doesn't help your child transition to independence. Every child is different; some may take longer to learn to go to sleep.

You know it's a problem when it is taking more than fifteen minutes for your child to fall asleep or they are waking one or more times during the night and need you to help them go back to sleep.

---

134 Owens and Mindell, *Take Charge of Your Child's Sleep.*

You may need to explore exactly why your child is anxious and having difficulty winding down. If you think the pattern is caused by behaviour and habit and you decide to change this pattern, a slow change will work the best.

Start by having cuddly time and 'kiss good night' time before they get into bed. Then, to break your pattern of lying down with them, start sitting in a chair next to them and make sure they have a special cuddly toy if they want one. As your child gets used to you in the chair, you can say to them, 'I'm leaving the room for two minutes and coming back in to say good night.' Do exactly as you have said, and this will leave them reassured that you are true to your word.

On successive nights, you could leave for longer periods and reward your child in the morning for staying super quiet and being a super sleeper by going to sleep on their own. Some parents find it helpful to slowly move their chair closer to the door on successive nights until the chair is sitting outside the child's room.

It will take time to break this pattern. At each stage, your child needs to feel reassured, safe and secure by you doing exactly what you said you would. They also need to follow the rules: no chatting, no excuses, no calling out. Once your child is going to sleep successfully on their own, middle-of-the-night waking will also be much easier to tackle because your child has learnt how to put him or herself back to sleep.

As always, if you suspect that the pattern is caused by more general anxiety or a sleep disorder, you will need to seek some expert help (see Chapter 6).

Night-time routine tips

Everyone experiences micro-arousals at night, during which we wake briefly but not fully. Most of us are unaware of waking. However, if a child requires help to go back to sleep, you have a night waking problem and need to come up with a good overnight routine to address it. A third of preschoolers wake up at least once a night and five per cent wake two or more times.[135]

Common causes of night waking are related to routine, environment, sleep disorders and behaviours. Routine-related causes might include a change to regular programming (such as being on holidays), a lack of firm rules and boundaries (so no routine) or having too many naps in the day. Environmental factors could include noise, temperature, comfort or a change in environment (such as a change of bedroom). Diagnosable sleep disorders can also lead to night waking – SDB, for instance, impacts sleep cycles by disrupting transition into the deep sleep component of stages 3 and 4, keeping them in lighter sleep phases where they are easily roused or disturbed. Finally, behavioural factors affecting night waking include being unwell or experiencing exciting or stressful daytime events that can lead to being wired or to scary nightmares.

A couple of years ago, a little three-year-old girl in my clinic came in visibly upset, and she could not settle to do our usual clinical activities. Eventually she crawled up on my lap and said that she was 'really scared from the yelling, and then a big storm came'. Her dad said nothing while I comforted the child and helped her talk about it. A couple of weeks later he divulged that the marriage had broken up. This little girl had real fears and needed comfort and nurturing to help her feel less afraid.

In many cases, overnight waking can be curbed by helping your child learn to put him or her self back to sleep once they wake. This follows naturally when they have learned to fall asleep on their own at the

135 Ibid.

beginning of the night, as described previously. If night waking and having help to resettle to sleep has been a habit, it may take a week or so of reassurance before your child is ready to do it alone. Gentle reassurance and a hug may be enough to encourage them back to sleep. Otherwise, repeating the initial bedtime strategy, blow by blow, will be helpful. This simply means you are using identical cues for the middle of the night as you did in the beginning. Eventually the need for your presence will fade, as it did for falling asleep in the beginning of the night. Cuddles and reassurance may be especially important if they have had a scary dream. In time, they will be able to follow the routine independently rather than waking up mum or dad to put them back to bed.

Here's a common conundrum. Many parents find a child who has crawled into bed next to them in the middle of the night. If they sleep quietly and do not move during sleep, then perhaps a parent's sleep will not be disturbed. While it is lovely to have those middle-of-the-night cuddles, it is not ideal if your sleep is disrupted and no one gets their correct quota of quality sleep. Conversely, if a parent is a restless or noisy sleeper, the child's sleep may be disrupted. What we are angling for is optimum sleep for everyone.

Note that 'waking' from sleep-walking or talking is a different matter. Kids experiencing parasomnias need to be directed calmly and quietly back to bed, and they will not recall any part of the walking or talking the next day. It's more frightening for parents, and of course you need to make sure your child is in no danger if wandering about the house, or worse, outside the house. Persistent parasomnias require medical advice.

GOING DEEPER: TO CO-SLEEP OR NOT TO CO-SLEEP

To co-sleep or not to co-sleep – that is the question. Stances on this issue vary culturally, with five- and six-year-old children still sleeping in their parents' bed in some Asian cultures, while many Western cultures have babies sleeping in a separate bassinet from birth.[136,137]

Medical advice may also influence parents' decisions about co-sleeping, as there are strict medical guidelines around babies and co-sleeping due to the higher likelihood of SIDS in a co-sleeping environment.[138]

Co-sleeping can become an issue if children have not learnt to settle themselves and if the reason for co-sleeping is a reactive attempt to solve sleep problems. As kids mature, it's important for kids to learn to put themselves to sleep, and back to sleep if they wake, thus learning independence.

However, if co-sleeping is part of your family philosophy, there is no reason to challenge this as long as everyone is getting the sleep they need. Be creative about how this can happen without disturbing sleep cycles. For example, have a mattress next to your bed where a child can sleep so that you will not disturb each other during wake-ups and movement – theirs or yours.

Whatever your decision, try to factor in the sleep formula and be confident that it poses no risk to safety, nor need it compromise the quantity and quality of everyone's sleep.

---

136 Sarah L. Blunden, 'Comment on: The Joy of Parenting: Infant Sleep Intervention to Improve Maternal Emotional Well-Being and Infant Sleep', *Singapore Medical Journal* 58, no. 3 (2017), https://doi.org/10.11622/smedj.2017019.

137 Sarah L. Blunden, Kirrilly R. Thompson and Drew Dawson, 'Behavioural Sleep Treatments and Night-Time Crying in Infants: Challenging the Status Quo', *Sleep Medicine Reviews* 15, no. 5 (2011), https://doi.org/10.1016/j.smrv.2010.11.002.

138 American Academy of Pediatrics, Task Force on Infant Sleep Position and Sudden Infant Death Syndrome, 'Changing Concepts of Sudden Infant Death Syndrome: Implications for Infant Sleeping Environment and Sleep Position', *Pediatrics* 105, no. 3 pt 1 (2000): 650–56.

Morning routine tips

It's important to go to bed at a consistent time with a consistent routine. It's just as important to wake up at the same time every day and follow a consistent morning routine.

Here are some tips to help kids wake up well:

- **Give a 'wake-up curfew' to early risers:** If your child can read a digital clock, you can teach them when they are allowed up by reading the number on the clock (it might need to say 7:00am, for example). It's also important to set rules around what they can do if they are up earlier than everyone else.

- **Wake kids up yourself:** Waking up to the soothing voice of mum or dad, perhaps with a little back rub, is a pleasant way for little ones to start the day.

- **Reward good sleep:** Morning is the perfect time to give rewards to kids who slept well the night before. Give them an instant positive cuddle and say how good they were for falling asleep so quickly. Praise and good moods are a great way to start the day, so find lots of little things to smile about.

- **Set the temperature:** Make sure the house is a comfortable temperature. If it's cold, have nice warm slippers and a dressing gown ready for your child to slip into.

- **Provide a nutritious breakfast:** Make sure there is yummy, nutritious food ready and available. For early risers, you could have some muesli bars or bananas in a bowl that they can easily reach. On a weekend, maybe you can provide breakfast in bed!

- **Get some sunlight:** Getting sunlight in the morning and during the day helps to reinforce the internal sleep-wake clock.[139]

- **Prepare for the day:** Talk about the day to come so your child knows what to expect and what to look forward to.

139 Stephen M. Pauley, 'Lighting for the Human Circadian Clock: Recent Research Indicates That Lighting Has Become a Public Health Issue', *Medical Hypotheses* 63, no. 4 (2004), https://doi.org/10.1016/j.mehy.2004.03.020.

It's important to be organised with your morning routine. This helps ensure that you aren't rushing around on work and school days and keeps the whole family calm and happy. Preparation the night before can help with this, such as laying out clothes for the next day. If mornings are tricky for your kids, a morning routine and a 'beat the buzzer game' may help motivate your kids to get ready for the day and be on time.

If your child has woken cranky and out of sorts, take a 'gently, gently' approach. Note that kids who have slept well should not wake up cranky or slowly on a regular basis. If your child has had the correct hours of sleep and is still waking up cranky, it's a red flag for poor sleep quality.

Daytime routine tips

Preparing for a good sleep starts with what you do in the day, as daytime behaviour problems are likely to lead to night-time shenanigans. Here are some things to keep in mind when it comes to your kids' daytime routines:

- **Napping schedule:** Daytime naps need to be carefully scheduled. If there's been a disruption to sleep due to a party or visitor, make sure you schedule a nap the next day, ensuring your child gets the correct number of hours sleep. (See Appendix A for some great tips about baby's naps from Tracy Newberry.)

- **Technology:** Increased technology use is eroding kids' sleep and leading to 'tech neck'. Screen use can cause overstimulation, add busyness to the daytime schedule and push out bedtimes – not to mention the interference with melatonin release caused by the blue light. Ensure that any use of screens is relaxing, and cut out daytime TV or particular shows if you think they are contributing to bedtime shenanigans. Screens should be off at least an hour before bed. (This advice is relevant for adults, too!)

- **Exercise:** Make sure your littlie has had good physical exercise and gets outside into the daylight. Ideally, running around and physical activity should wind down a couple of hours before bed.

- **Nutrition:** Make sure your kids are eating regular meals and snacks, 'as close to nature as possible' – predominantly healthy, unprocessed foods without additives and sugar. It's important your child has enough iron as well as the vitamins and minerals found in fresh fruit and vegetables, such as vitamins A, D and K. There are some great resources on nutrition, and involving kids in food preparation and making it fun can also make a huge difference to their attitude with food.[140,141,142]

- **Busy mind:** Engage your child's brain during the day with puzzle books and activities like cooking rather than passive activities like watching TV. Also, tune into whether they are worried about anything – you can talk through the worry, or help them visualise taking the worry out of their head and putting it 'in the bin with a lid on'.

140 Steven Lin, *The Dental Diet: The Surprising Link Between Your Teeth, Real Food, and Life-Changing Natural Health* (Carlsbad, CA: Hay House, Inc., 2018).

141 Max Lugavere, *Genius Foods: Become Smarter Happier and More Productive while Protecting Your Brain for Life* (Harper Collins, NY: 2018)

142 Bill and Claire Wurtzel, *Funny Food: 365 Fun, Healthy, Silly Creative Breakfasts* (Welcome Enterprises, NY: 2012)

ROUTINES FOR KIDS WITH ADHD

For children with ADHD, it's critical to start the pre-sleep slowdown period early afternoon and evening in order to minimise sleep disturbances. Alongside this, you'll want to develop strategies to cope with anxiety, build positive sleep associations and instil good sleep habits.

But even with good bedtime routines, kids with ADHD can have trouble switching off their thinking and winding down their bodies from the happenings and activities of the day. Switching off thoughts and winding down 'overdrive' is different to the healthy brain activity that happens in restorative sleep. Events that may have revved up or upset your child will impact their ability to calm down before bed, exacerbated by their challenges with emotional self-regulation. Of course, being overtired exacerbates everything. This can be confusing with such kids because they appear to be energetic, when really they are wired-tired.

I met parents recently whose nine-year-old child with ADHD had become very wired and anxious. They said it was so difficult to get the daytime school events under control that they started home-schooling. This eliminated a lot of the social anxiety he was experiencing, which helped him settle far better for bed – even though he still goes to bed later than ideal. This may be in part due to the medication he is taking for his ADHD. They are now able to let him sleep in to ensure that he gets the total correct number of hours of sleep because he doesn't need to get up for school. It has made a huge difference for him – and them.

Some strategies that may help kids with ADHD include adjusting timing of medications that may exacerbate sleep difficulties, using incentives, and adjusting their bedtimes to account for their alert periods. If all else fails, your doctor may suggest a sleep helper medication and perhaps recommend further professional help for emotional and psychological issues.

Helping new routines stick

Having covered the changes you can make to bedtime, night-time and daytime routines, you are probably ready to implement a number of changes for your child. At this point, I'll repeat my earlier advice about implementing changes: make only a few changes at a time, don't negotiate on them and be consistent and patient.

Here are a few more suggestions about how to help routine changes stick. These will be particularly helpful for toddlers, who need that bit of extra parental guidance to try new things.

- **Explain how things will work:** It doesn't work well for young kids to have new things simply sprung on them. When you explain things, focus on the positive (what to do) not on the negative (what not to do). Desirable behaviours are easier to get going when framed in a positive way. For example, using phrases like 'going to bed happy, staying super quiet, staying super still and going to sleep super-fast (or becoming a super sleeper)' is much more effective than telling toddlers not to make noise. Kids respond to this approach amazingly well and are very proud of being super sleepers.

- **Give your kids choice:** You can make your toddler's bedtime routine more enjoyable by letting them have a choice of activities before bed. For example, would they like a story or a meditation tonight? You can also make a set of routine cards, or buy pre-prepared ones, that represent each stage of your routine, ideally with pictures, and your child can choose which one they want to do each night.

- **Use visual supports:** Kids respond very well to visuals, so consider creating a visual chart with each of your child's bedtime routine activities where they get a star for each one as it's completed. Or you can make a set of routine cards that represent each stage of your morning or evening routine, and your child places the routine card into a 'posting box' as each part of the routine is done. Kids learn a routine very quickly, especially with visual supports, and they may be able to tell you what's next or let you know when a part of the routine is not necessary. You can even make a Kanban board for your morning and bedtime routines.[143] Kids' Kanban is adapted from the original text by Benson and DeMaria Barry, and a book on kids Kanban by DeMaria is coming out soon. Children can help make sticky notes to represent each part of the bedtime routine and move sticky notes to the 'done' column when done. The sensory input from touching, feeling and moving the sticky notes gives kids a great sense of achievement that comes from a completed task. The visuals also reinforce memory of the routine and make each night successively easier.

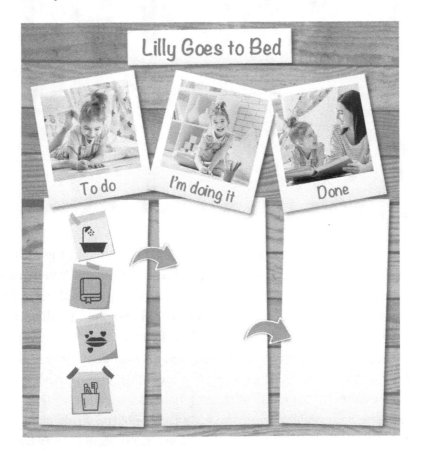

143 Jim Benson and Tonianne De Maria. Barry, *Personal Kanban: Mapping Work, Navigating Life* (Seattle, WA: Modus Cooperandi Press, 2011).

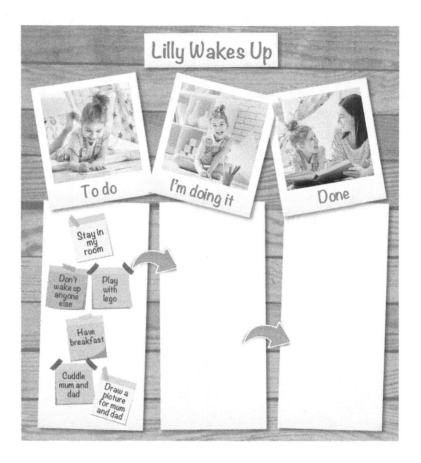

- **Use rewards**. For many kids, little tangible rewards for their efforts work well, like stamps on a chart, stickers or balloons. You can also build up to bigger rewards if they do all activities without a fuss or do them for several nights in a row. Kids respond to all sorts of rewards: you can start with a small daily incentive: 'When you get to sleep super fast and you have posted all your cards, you will find a little surprise in your room in the morning'. End-of-week incentives can really help kids with long haul sleep issues, as they help to create your daily routine and give a sense of the week, especially if they can see a weekly calendar and see their progress day by day. For some, an experience like going to a movie will motivate them: 'If you post all your cards every night Monday through to Friday, we can go to a movie on Saturday.' Ticks and stickers also work well as incentives for many kids as does a coin jar. Other kids will enjoy something like dressing up in a favourite hat or costume all day. Incentivising with a weekly reward once your day-to-day routine is working can come in many different forms to suit your family style.

Be consistent with rewards, as they only work if they are applied as promised. If the agreed behaviour is achieved, the reward is given. If was not achieved, there is no surprise. Some parents don't like to use rewards, as they are concerned that it will set up long-term expectations by a child, thinking that rewards will be expected for every single aspect of getting cooperation. This happens only if rewards are being used for *everything*. The system suggested here is for a single behaviour and short-term use. If rewards are being used for every aspect of a child's life that is a red flag for professional intervention.

Most children really want to please mum and dad. As children learn the consequences of what they say and do, little rewards for managing change and following directions that help with bedtime, overnight or morning routines can be great habit-changing helpers. For many kids, seeing the smile on mum and dad's face or receiving cuddles from pleased parents is enough reward.

Finally, keep tabs on progress and celebrate the wins. Perhaps have a calendar on the wall so that your child can see their progress. Keep in mind that success may not be immediate. Changing habits and creating new ones takes time. You need to hang in there – be consistent and persistent and, if you stick to it like glue for at least two weeks, most kids settle really well.

But if you're finding it hard to get those new habits bedded down (pun intended!) then I have one more suggestion for you.

Third-party magic

After decades of working with children and their families who want to create new habits and extinguish old ones, I have observed that families face a few challenges that can get in the way. Common issues I see are resistance from children, inconsistency from parents and conflict. The end result is not behaviour change but a pattern of failed attempts – in other words, a 'failure cycle'. Some of this is because children have an uncanny ability to press their parents' buttons, tug at their heartstrings in ways that undermine parental consistency, making behaviour change very difficult. It's also hard to be persistent. Let's face it; life is full of demands. I have frequently watched on as parents try out a new approach, only to give up on it if the approach takes effort or doesn't work immediately. Then they will try something different, lack persistence and pull out, resulting in an entrenched pattern of failure that can be hard to break. The end result is frayed nerves, sometimes damaged relationships, no behaviour change and, worst of all, a lack of hope.

After many years of helping kids to change habits like thumb-sucking, I realised that a key factor to success was the child's accountability to me instead of their parents. Parents agree with this. The systems I used were positive and rewards based to keep kids motivated and on track, and I was 'unbending' about rules. Firm and kind is the motto. I therefore began to apply the same principles to sleep issues. This is how 'third-party magic' developed, and it is still used successfully to this day in my clinic. Kids happily follow the rules I set, and if they lapse they get back on track very quickly.

Third-party magic works really well. But to be able to help a lot more kids without always being physically present with them, I have developed various characters to help parents use this third-party concept at home, enabling a sense of accountability without me being directly involved. One such character is Granny Twinkle, a grandmother character I've developed. Granny Twinkle has helped parents 'sweep the room' for monsters, but Granny Twinkle can help with many other things in the routine. For example, with bespoke routine cards, Granny Twinkle might be the person behind the routine instructions: 'Granny Twinkle says it's time to brush your teeth'; 'Granny Twinkle said you can have one tick for doing your teeth without a fuss, two ticks if your teeth look sparkly and clean'; 'Granny Twinkle says you can choose a story or mini yoga, which one do you choose?'; 'Granny Twinkle says use the silver magic spray to help all your teddies fall asleep.' The possibilities are endless. This creative world is so much fun for kids.

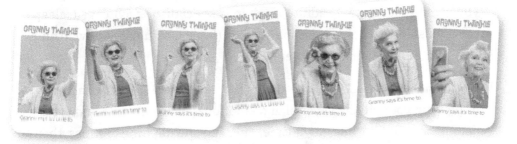

A character like Granny Twinkle may be able to provide enough of the third-party magic to assist you in establishing new, healthy patterns. But if it's not enough, then it might be worth enlisting the help of a physical third party to break these unhelpful habits. When bedtime has become a battleground, chances are there may be other battlegrounds in your child's daily life as well. That's when calling in a third party can be really helpful as it defuses the conflict between parents and children while you are settling new habits and routines (especially when every-one is tired, which can be a recipe for escalating tension). Resolving the battlegrounds in daily life can resolve sleep battles as well. For some families, a friend or family member may be able to perform this defus-ing role. Third-party magic can be helpful with 'real people' as well, not just fictional characters.

Sometimes a change in environment is the best way to break a habit. Try having an aunt, uncle or grandparent come over to put the kids to bed for a few nights while mum and dad go on a short holiday, or try sending the kids for a sleepover at a relative's house for a few nights. As long as the third party on hand knows the right routine and does not respond to the child's usual delay tactics and bedtime shenanigans, this approach can work wonders. Once the new routine is set outside home, the next step is to reinforce the new routine back at home. It may be that an aunty can come and help at home for a couple of nights to kick start the new habit. Remember, when it's your turn to follow the routine as parents, follow it to the letter, or it won't work.

However, if stalling behaviour is causing family conflict and tension and you can't find a suitable adult to step in, a specialist psychologist, sleep coach or sleep nanny may be able to help. (We'll look more at how to find the right expert help in Chapter 6.)

If you manage to address the things we've covered in this chapter by improving your child's physical and emotional environments and establishing healthy bedtime, night-time, morning and daytime routines, then your child's sleep will improve beyond measure – along with your own.

However, if you've done it all and there are still some red flags popping up, then it's time to look deeper. In this case, the issues causing your child's sleeping difficulties might be physical, not behavioural. We're going to look at that next. Just like lifesavers train the little nippers how to be strong swimmers, being a lifeguard for your child's airway will help them have optimal breathing and better quality sleep.

CHAPTER FIVE

How to build a healthy airway, the 'myo' way

Healthy sleep requires a healthy airway. You can create the perfect environment and stick to textbook routines, but if your child can't breathe well then their sleep quality will suffer.

But isn't the health of our airway just the luck of genetics? In the minds of many, we're born with the physical features we have. Our airway setup, and our child's airway health, simply is what it is, right?

Actually, you have far more influence over the shape and development of your child's airway health than you might believe. This is both a big responsibility and a big relief, as it means that there's hope to change even the most challenging physical issues that could be impeding good, healthy breathing and sleep quality.

When the muscles of the mouth, face and throat develop poorly or develop poor habits, children may experience sleep-disordered breathing. The muscles we use for sucking, swallowing, breathing and chewing – especially how they are used and developed in our early years – can have a big impact on breathing during sleep, and subsequently on sleep quality.[144] Similarly, the structure and shape of the face and jaws also have an impact on sleep breathing and quality. Our jaws rely on optimal muscle function to grow and develop. For this reason, it's important to make sure that littlies learn how to use these muscles correctly.[145] If this sub-optimal muscles use is not fully treated, sleep-disordered breathing can persist or recur throughout life.

---

144 Guilleminault and Huang, 'From Oral Facial Dysfunction to Dysmorphism and the Onset Of Pediatric OSA'.

145 Christian Guilleminault, 'A Case for Myofunctional Therapy as a Standard of Care for Pediatric OSA', in *The 2nd AAMS Congress* (Chicago, 2017).

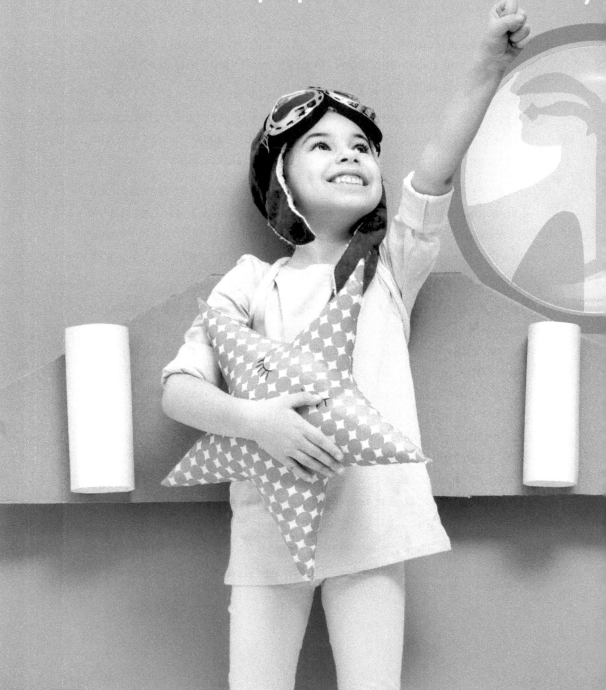

Factors which
upper airway

mpact a child's development

Underlying genetics

How the muscles of the face mouth and throat are used (from birth) including posture

Epigenetics (environment and lifestyle factors)

Health status and immunity

Healthy gestation

The role of myofunctional therapy

This is where myofunctional (myo) health comes in. Let's start with health, *orofacial myofunctional health*. What a mouthful! What does this mean?

'Orofacial' refers to the mouth and face. 'Myo' means muscle, and 'function' refers to the way the system works. 'Health' then refers to whether the system is healthy, working at its optimum and exactly as it should for the functions it is required to do. The functions are the very things we do all day every day to sustain our body, things like swallowing, breathing, eating and drinking. We rarely turn our attention to what our tongue and lips do while we are chewing, nor do we think about how we breathe. We eat for pleasure and hunger. We breathe to stay alive, and it just happens, right? Well, yes. However, to create a pro-active mindset to healthy function, awareness is key. Poor habits can develop easily without us even knowing, and what if the wrong kind of habits have developed (the ones that impede healthy function), how would you know? That's where the pro-active approach to myo comes in.

Myo is a therapeutic technique used to educate or re-educate the oral and facial muscles for optimal breathing, sucking, facial muscle movement, eating and drinking – in other words, to get them all working well as a system, eliminating harmful habits and correcting problems. Myo also establishes ideal 'rest' postures for the muscles, meaning where the muscles sit when they have nothing else to do. Establishing correct myo habits as early as possible makes a big difference to airway health and sleep quality. Why? Because healthy muscle function influences bone growth and specifically jaw growth, which are foundation structures of the airway.

Promoting myo health usually starts with exercises for the tongue, lips, cheeks, jaws and throat, and head and neck posture. This muscle re-education leads on to optimising the way the muscles are used in daily life for the essential life functions of breathing and eating which will impact not only airway patency (which means 'degree of openness') but also the other functions of the upper airway like speaking and vocalising. Yes, lots of things happen in the upper airway. Optimising these muscle functions promotes healthy bone growth and can minimise the effect of medical issues that lead to a small or narrow airway, or conditions that lead to weak or poorly coordinated muscles in the airway. Lifelong upper airway health is essential to our physical, mental, emotional and social capability.

A myofunctional assessment examines the face, mouth and throat from three different perspectives: how it looks, how it sounds, how it works. The assessment pinpoints any issues with size and shape of the structures, and how the system functions for everyday activities and where muscles rest habitually. Both daytime and night-time aspects are taken into account in the assessment. To diagnose a myofunctional disorder of the mouth, face and throat, we look at:

- Muscle rest postures
- Muscle movement patterns: breathing, chewing, swallowing and speech
- Oral habits

Then we look at factors that influence, or are associated with, those functions:

- The size, shape and structure of the face and upper airway passages
- The health of the soft tissues in the face and upper airway
- Any contributing medical, dental or orthodontic concern
- Any contributing early developmental challenge

Any functional problem diagnosed is known as an *orofacial myofunctional disorder*. This refers to any dysfunction of any part of the upper airway, extending from the front of the face all the way to the voice box or larynx, which may occur or exist in conjunction with or resulting from discrepancies with the shape or size of the bony structures of the face. For example, if the upper jaw is very narrow, it may be difficult for the tongue to rest in its ideal position. If the upper jaw shape has been distorted by a thumb or finger sucking habit, the tongue rest posture is altered and may sit forward as an adaption to the altered shape of the upper jaw and teeth.

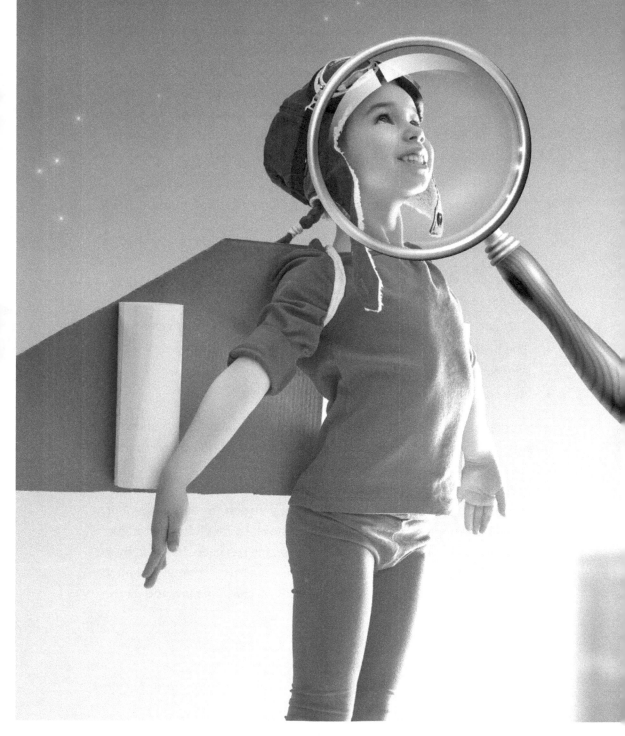

What does **orofacia**

myofunctional mean?

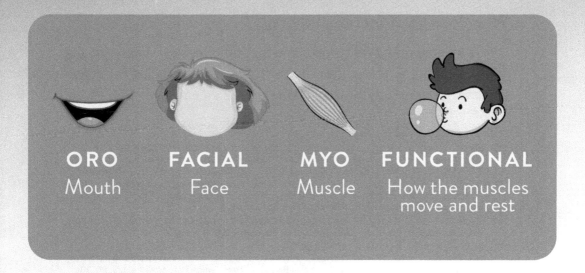

ORO
Mouth

FACIAL
Face

MYO
Muscle

FUNCTIONAL
How the muscles
move and rest

Multiple studies have shown that myo exercises for the upper airway can reduce the severity of OSA and SDB.[146,147,148,149,150,151,152] Myofunctional therapy has been shown to reduce snoring in adults and has even been shown to improve the efficacy of CPAP treatment.[153,154] Dr Maria Pia Villa et al published a paper in 2017 showing that exercises for the mouth and back of the throat were effective for modifying tongue tone, reducing SDB symptoms and mouth breathing and improving oxygen saturation in breathing.[155]

Who does myofunctional therapy?

Myo is an emerging field of medicine that functions as a sub-specialty within existing health professions such as speech pathology or dental hygiene. It is important to know that myo is an emerging field rather

146 Macario Camacho, Victor Certal, Jose Abdullatif, Soroush Zaghi, Chad M. Ruoff, Robson Capasso and Clete A. Kushida, 'Myofunctional Therapy to Treat Obstructive Sleep Apnea: A Systematic Review and Meta-analysis', *Sleep* 38, no. 5 (2015), https://doi.org/10.5665/sleep.4652.

147 Camila De Castro Corrêa and Giédre Berretin-Felix, 'Terapia miofuncional orofacial aplicada à Síndrome do aumento da resistência das vias aéreas superiores: caso clínico', *CoDAS* 27, no. 6 (2015), https://doi.org/10.1590/2317-1782/20152014228.

148 Nicole Archambault Besson, 'The Tongue Was Involved, but What Was the Trouble?' *ASHA Leader* 20, no. 9 (2015), https://doi.org/10.1044/leader.cp.20092015.np.

149 Kátia C. Guimarães, Luciano F. Drager, Pedro R. Genta, Bianca F. Marcondes and Geraldo Lorenzi-Filh, 'Effects of Oropharyngeal Exercises on Patients with Moderate Obstructive Sleep Apnea Syndrome', *American Journal of Respiratory and Critical Care Medicine* 179, no. 10 (2009), https://doi.org/10.1164/rccm.200806-981oc.

150 Giovana Diaferia, Luciana Badke, Rogerio Santos-Silva, Silvana Bommarito, Sergio Tufik and Lia Bittencourt, 'Effect of Speech Therapy as Adjunct Treatment to Continuous Positive Airway Pressure on the Quality of Life of Patients with Obstructive Sleep Apnea', *Sleep Medicine* 14, no. 7 (2013), https://doi.org/10.1016/j.sleep.2013.03.016.

151 C. Guilleminault, Y. S. Huang, P. J. Monteyrol, R. Sato, S. Quo and C.H. Lin, 'Critical Role of Myofascial Reeducation in Pediatric Sleep-Disordered Breathing', *Sleep Medicine* 14, no. 6 (2013), https://doi.org/10.1016/j.sleep.2013.01.013.

152 Huang and Guilleminault, 'Pediatric Obstructive Sleep Apnea and the Critical Role of Oral-Facial Growth: Evidences'.

153 Macario Camacho, Christian Guilleminault, Justin M. Wei, Sungjin A. Song, Michael W. Noller, Lauren K. Reckley, Camilo Fernandez-Salvador and Soroush Zaghi, 'Oropharyngeal and Tongue Exercises (Myofunctional Therapy) for Snoring: A Systematic Review and Meta-Analysis', *European Archives of Oto-Rhino-Laryngology*, 2017, https://doi.org/10.1007/s00405-017-4848-5.

154 Diaferia et al., 'Effect of Speech Therapy as Adjunct Treatment to Continuous Positive Airway Pressure'.

155 Maria Pia Villa, Melania Evangelisti, Susy Martella, Mario Barreto and Marco Del Pozzo, 'Can Myofunctional Therapy Increase Tongue Tone and Reduce Symptoms in Children with Sleep-Disordered Breathing?' *Sleep and Breathing* 21, no. 4 (2017), https://doi.org/10.1007/s11325-017-1489-2.

>> it's still a largely unknown field to many health practitioners as well as to the parents and children who could benefit from it most

than a fully established discipline, and further studies are required[156] to fully establish its scope of practice and role in medicine. Its benefits are starting to gain global traction but it's still a largely unknown field to many health practitioners as well as to the parents and children who could benefit from it the most. This is, of course, one of the reasons I've written this book – to demonstrate just how beneficial myofunctional therapy can be for sleep-wrecked kids and their sleep-deprived parents!

While myo is not a replacement for medical treatment when needed, it is the perfect therapy to use alongside medical and dental treatments to reinforce, rehabilitate and maintain orofacial health.[157,158,159]

Myo and sleep disorders

When things go wrong with upper airway and affect sleep, a medical or dental opinion is important. However, many kids slip under the radar and may be first identified by another allied health practitioner, such as an occupational therapist, physiotherapist, psychologist,

156 Fabiane Kayamori and Esther Mandelbaum Gonçalves Bianchini, 'Effects of Orofacial Myofunctional Therapy on the Symptoms and Physiological Parameters of Sleep Breathing Disorders in Adults: A Systematic Review', *Revista* CEFAC 19, no. 6 (2017), https://doi.org/10.1590/1982-0216201719613317.

157 Yasuyo Sugawara, Yoshihito Ishihara, Teruko Takano-Yamamoto, Takashi Yamashiro and Hiroshi Kamioka, 'Orthodontic Treatment of a Patient with Unilateral Orofacial Muscle Dysfunction: The Efficacy of Myofunctional Therapy on the Treatment Outcome', *American Journal of Orthodontics and Dentofacial Orthopedics* 150, no. 1 (2016), https://doi.org10.1016/j.ajodo.2015.08.021.

158 S. Saccomanno, G. Antonini, L. D'Alatri, M. D'Angelantonio, A. Fiorita and R. Deli, 'Causal Relationship Between Malocclusion and Oral Muscles Dysfunction: A Model of Approach', *Eur J Paediatr Dent* 13, no. 4 (2012): 321–23.

159 Joann Smithpeter and David Covell, 'Relapse of Anterior Open Bites Treated with Orthodontic Appliances with and without Orofacial Myofunctional Therapy', *American Journal of Orthodontics and Dentofacial Orthopedics* 137, no. 5 (2010), https://doi.org/10.1016/j.ajodo.2008.07.016.

speech pathologist or myofunctional practitioner. Any allied health practitioners who see children of all ages, including babies, are in the front line.[160] They are perfectly positioned to call attention to myofunctional red flags and also upper airway problems. You could argue that all allied health practitioners have an ethical responsibility to recognise such red flags.

There is growing recognition for the use of myo worldwide, with a groundswell of sleep specialists recommending myofunctional therapy as an adjunctive treatment option for airway related sleep disorders. The Brazilian Sleep Society was the first national medical society to adopt myo as a standard of medical care in sleep disorders with airway obstruction, with twenty-three speech pathologists in Brazil credentialed in 2018 to work with sleep disorders and ever-increasing numbers.

>> **The American Pediatric Association released a key action statement saying that all clinicians should screen for sleep-disordered breathing**

The French Society of Research and Sleep Medicine announced myofunctional therapy as an adjunctive standard of care in paediatric OSA. The Asian Paediatric Pulmonary Society has also adopted myo as a standard of care with paediatric sleep apnoea.[161] The American Academy of Orthodontics has also acknowledged the role of myofunctional practice in developing and maintaining dental and occlusal health. Moreover, The American Pediatric Association released a key action statement saying all clinicians should screen for SDB.

In his 2017 presentation at the AAMS Workshop World Sleep Society Conference in Prague, Dr Stanley Liu said, 'Myofunctional therapy is the missing link in sleep surgery. Surgery can decrease the severity level of

160 Moore, 'Sleep Disorders are in Your Face'.
161 'The Asian Paediatric Pulmonology Society (APPS) Position Statement on Childhood Obstructive Sleep Apnea Syndrome', *Erratum* 1, no. 3 (2017): 69, https://doi.org/10.4103/WKMP-0132.216541.

OSA but it always relapses. There is a place for myofunctional therapy in every phase of sleep surgery.'[162]

If you or your health practitioner have identified any early red flags for sleep-disordered breathing, or you want to be proactive before any problems become worse or develop into habits, it's time to see how myo can help.

Optimising sleep with myo

In my clinic, I have developed and recommend two therapeutic approaches: *myo-optimise* and *myo-correct*. In this chapter, we'll be looking at the myo-optimise approach for ways that you can work, either on your own or with a practitioner, to optimise airway health for your child. We will address myo-correct, which focusses more on assessment, diagnosis and treatment for *myofunctional disorders, later in this chapter*.

>> Myo can benefit every child well before any sleep breathing disorder develops or nip any early signs in the bud.

Myo-optimise involves optimising the muscles from birth (or even in-utero) so that the face, mouth and throat all develop to their best potential from the earliest possible age. Myo can benefit every child well before any sleep breathing disorder develops or nip any early signs in the bud. This is a pro-active approach to address a major public health issue. The general principles and ways of using the muscles can be taught and encouraged from day one of a baby's life, and every day thereafter. In ideal conditions, myo-optimisation is done by the time a child is six years old (before their first adult teeth appear and before they start school), as this capitalises on a young child's extraordinary capacity

---

162 Stanley Liu, 'From Reconstruction to Re-Education: The Evolution of a Sleep Surgery Protocol with DOME, MMA, Hypoglossal Nerve Stimulation, and Myofunctional Therapy', AAMS Workshop, pre *World Sleep Society Conference* (Prague, 2017).

for growth and change and sets them up with good habits rather than having to correct bad habits. Good muscle function encourages good bone growth. Whilst early is best and it is easier to develop good habits than undo bad ones, change can happen at any age, so it's never too late to start. Myo-optimise is a corrective strategy and a preventive approach rolled into one.

Before starting any myo program, it may be helpful to start with an individual assessment to see if your child is suitable for an optimisation or correction program. From there, an individual program can be designed, specific to their needs, aiming for optimal function as early as possible in a child's life.

In this chapter, I'm going to teach you the basic approach of myofunctional therapy so that you're equipped to start supporting and optimising your child's airway health. Even if you don't undertake any formal myofunctional therapy, you will learn a lot and be able to apply much of it simply by reading about the myo-optimise approach.

No matter the age of your child, whether you have a baby, school age child or you intend to have more children in the future, this information will be particularly applicable for you and will empower you in your role as life-guard. You'll be able to shape your child's airway health to a great degree. For those of you with older kids who may feel that they have missed the boat on myo-optimisation, don't despair – it is never too late. For teenagers, myo issues tend to be much more like adult issues, but the same principles apply. Myo can be undertaken throughout life. You may even discover that you have airway issues or habits yourself and will benefit from doing the exercises. In fact, in clinic, we always encourage a whole family approach.

The ideal scenario is when the whole family gets on board and does the program. I am constantly amazed at how much fun these activities can be, especially when the whole family is participating. In my clinic, the age-specific programs contain motivating games and rewards that are suited to different age groups. Many parents I see are really clever

>> **The whole focus is to have fun and integrate the activities into your daily life so they become natural and are not a chore**

at adapting programs to the home environment. The whole focus is to have fun and integrate the activities into your daily life so they become natural and are not a chore.

So, you don't have to go to clinic to get an optimise program going. The main point here is more about the ultimate goal, and that whatever you are doing is helping to achieve your goals. However, if there is a diagnosable problem then it is better to enlist in an intensive myo-correct program (see Chapter 6).

Myo-optimise: How to prepare your kids for good airway from day one

Myo-optimise is an approach designed to capitalise on establishing good myo habits for young children. When looking at myofunctional health of the upper airway, we consider how things are developing from the very beginning, with optimising goals in mind for the following stages:

1. In utero
2. While breastfeeding
3. During nose breathing
4. When transitioning to solids
5. While learning to talk
6. During games to promote good airway
7. While muscles are at rest

Getting things right from day one may be simple, but it isn't always easy – there's a lot to keep an eye on and be aware of. We'll address each of these areas one by one, looking first at what needs to happen for optimal development and what can get in the way, then looking at what you can do to ensure great upper airway health in your child.

>> Believe it or not, healthy sleep starts while a baby is still in mum's tummy

In utero

Believe it or not, healthy sleep starts while a baby is still in mum's tummy. The way babies learn to use the muscles for sucking and swallowing in utero, and subsequently in the very early years, is the beginning of healthy development of the jaws and upper airway, essential for good sleep.[163]

How so?

By the twentieth week of pregnancy, the part of the early embryo that develops into the mouth grows, allowing the tongue and mouth cavity to develop. From the twentieth week, the tongue grows and develops control from the brainstem and the baby should be actively sucking and swallowing from the third trimester. Three months of sucking and swallowing in utero prepares the baby for sucking and swallowing at birth. It also helps widen the upper jaw and stimulate growth of the lower jaw.

Although actual breathing does not happen in utero, around nine weeks into the pregnancy your baby makes breathing-like movements. Lung development begins early in pregnancy but is not complete until the third trimester, which is when the lungs develop alveoli, the tiny lung sacs that fill with oxygen, allowing your baby to take its first real breath at birth. From then on, nose breathing with the tongue resting on the palate helps to stimulate growth of the upper jaw. In a baby's tiny mouth, the tongue fills the oral cavity and rests beautifully up on the palate if it is a nice broad shape. The tongue resting on the palate helps to maintain the broad flat shape of the palate.

If a mother experiences sleep-disordered breathing and other health issues during pregnancy, it can interfere with myofunctional development

---

163 Guilleminault and Huang, 'From Oral Facial Dysfunction to Dysmorphism and the Onset Of Pediatric OSA'.

in utero.[164] We all know how smoking causes hypoxia and that smoking during pregnancy deprives the developing baby of critical oxygen, leading to low birth weight and other problems. What may surprise you is that your own sleep-breathing issues can also affect your baby while you are pregnant, by compromising delivery of oxygen to you and your baby.[165]

There is growing data on pregnant women to indicate that SDB, snoring and OSA increase the risk of preeclampsia, gestational diabetes and other complications for the mother and the baby that can lead to premature birth.[166] As pregnancy progresses, existing SDB worsens. Nasal congestion increases with weight gain, in turn increasing the risk of high blood pressure.[167] Pregnant women with hypertension are also at high risk for unrecognised OSA, which can then further promote hypertension.[168] A mother's health, compromised by sleep disorders that contribute to high blood pressure, may lead to premature birth via induction (due to doctors being concerned about slowed foetal movement) and the baby may not be mature enough to manage good breastfeeding.

Premature infants miss out on some essential third trimester suck-swallow training, which is why they can have problems establishing strong, well-coordinated feeding. If breastfeeding is not possible because of this, it means babies miss further suck-swallow training and early jaw development. This can be compounded by immature lungs in babies born prior to thirty-eight weeks. Missing essential suck-swallow

164 Anilawan Smitthimedhin, Matthew Whitehead, Mahya Bigdeli, Nino Gustavo, Perez Geovanny and Otero Hansel, 'MRI Determination of Volumes for the Upper Airway and Pharyngeal Lymphoid Tissue in Preterm and Term Infants', Clinical Imaging 50 (2018), https://doi.org/10.1016/j.clinimag.2017.12.010.

165 L. M. Obrien, A. S Bullough, M. C Chames, A. V Shelgikar, R. Armitage, C. Guilleminault, C. E. Sullivan, T. Johnson, and R. D. Chervin, 'Hypertension, Snoring, and Obstructive Sleep Apnoea During Pregnancy: A Cohort Study', BJOG: An International Journal of Obstetrics & Gynaecology 121, no. 13 (2014), https://doi.org/10.1111/1471-0528.12885.

166 Bilgay Izci-Balserak and Grace W. Pien, 'Sleep-Disordered Breathing and Pregnancy: Potential Mechanisms and Evidence for Maternal and Fetal Morbidity', Current Opinion in Pulmonary Medicine 16, no. 6 (2010), https://doi.org/10.1097/mcp.0b013e32833f0d55.

167 Amy Corderoy, 'Late-Pregnancy Snoring Risk To Baby: Study', Sydney Morning Herald, October 27, 2011, http://www.smh.com.au/national/health/latepregnancy-snoring-risk-to-baby-study-20111026-1mk9q.html.

168 Obrien et al., 'Hypertension, Snoring, and Obstructive Sleep Apnoea During Pregnancy: A Cohort Study'.

training then can mean a weaker suck, poorer coordination and, ultimately, challenges in breathing, breastfeeding and even bottle-feeding. The baby misses the early muscle stimulation for bone growth, which is a poor start for the early development of bones in the face and mouth.

WHAT YOU CAN DO

What is the best way to help babies move well and get the important practice of sucking and swallowing before birth while in utero?

If you are a mother, then it comes back to taking care of *your* health first. A mother's health has a big impact on the way a baby develops, its neural maturity at birth, and its readiness and ability to feed and breathe well. It's one long chain reaction, so when doctors are drawing attention to nutrition, hydration and breathing for pregnant mothers, it is a big deal. And it's important to make corrections as early as possible to give your baby the best chance of going to full term.

>> Snoring and OSA in pregnant women deprives the baby of oxygen

Snoring and OSA in pregnant women deprives the baby of oxygen. This causes your baby to move less in the womb, including doing less of the essential sucking, swallowing and breathing movements that prepare the baby for feeding and breathing well at birth.

By contrast, when you are healthy, your unborn baby makes the appropriate muscle movements of the mouth, face and throat in utero, preparing them for effective breastfeeding at birth.

Therefore, caring for your baby's health starts with you caring for your own health (in this case, particularly if you're the mother). This means ensuring you are a healthy weight, getting enough exercise, managing your stress and eating well. Minimising exposure to pollutants is also a factor. If you don't sleep well due to upper airway issues of your own, you can consult a GP or ear, nose and throat specialist about ensuring you can breathe easily through your nose. If you have more serious breathing issues, see a sleep specialist so you can breathe well at night. I also recommend Dr Steven Park's podcast *Breathe Better, Sleep Better, Live Better* for information on how to be proactive with your upper airway health.[169]

If your baby is born premature or is not breastfeeding well, there are exercises mums can do with bubs to stimulate the muscle movements required for feeding, including use of the baby's natural reflexes. Kick-starting their system via myofunctional or oro-motor therapy is key, in conjunction with essential medical supports.[170] I suggest taking a look at the approach taught by Debra Beckman.[171]

Breastfeeding

From birth until the first adult teeth come in around age six, the sutures of the palate (the soft segments that join the upper jaw bones together) are at their softest, most flexible and moveable. In fact, the upper jaw has connections to multiple other bones of the head and face. And because muscle function impacts the growth and development of many bones joined by sutures, the best time to influence that growth and development is in the very beginning when the sutures are at their softest. The movement of the tongue, cheeks and lips, which are all used for sucking during breastfeeding, contribute to face, mouth and jaw growth. Facial bone development is at its maximum growth rate from birth to the age of two, and there is much parents can do to help this process.

First, it's important to stimulate the palate through strong tongue movement against the palate and the gums surrounding the baby's teeth

---

169 Steven Y. Park, 'Breathe Better, Sleep Better, Live Better Podcast', podcast, https://itunes.apple.com/us/podcast/id292095799.

170 Brenda S. Lessen, 'Effect of the Premature Infant Oral Motor Intervention on Feeding Progression and Length of Stay in Preterm Infants', *Advances in Neonatal Care* 11, no. 2 (2011), https://doi.org/10.1097/anc.0b013e3182115a2a.

171 You can find Debra Beckman's work at https://www.beckmanoralmotor.com.

>> **The phrase 'breast is best' refers not just to the nutritional benefits of breast milk but also to the way breastfeeding establishes foundation muscle movement patterns that stimulate jaw growth and optimal airway development**

buds. For the first six months of life, this stimulation occurs mostly with breastfeeding. The phrase 'breast is best' refers not just to the nutritional benefits of breast milk but also to the way breastfeeding establishes foundation muscle movement patterns that stimulate jaw growth and optimal airway development.

As a baby grows, the structure of their face and mouth changes, and is influenced by feeding method and position. Muscle movement also adapts and changes in response to factors like milk flow and feeding position. An upright or semi-upright position is preferred as it encourages the tongue up into the palate during breastfeeding and helps keep it in a broad, flat shape, which encourages nose breathing (more on this later). Diane Bahr is a great resource for this, and I highly recommend her books, *Nobody Ever Told Me (Or My Mother) That!: Everything from Bottles and Breathing to Healthy Speech Development* and *How to Feed Your Baby and Toddler Right*.[172]

Efficient breastfeeding requires a good lip and cheek seal and full insertion of the breast into the baby's mouth. The back of the tongue lowers to create a vacuum that draws milk out of the breast and into the oesophagus. The vacuum action then creates a lot of activity on the back of throat, thought to be a key factor in keeping baby's ear tubes nice and open. Having the muscle systems working at their best is also good for ear drainage, as the middle ear tubes, also called the Eusta-

---

172 Diane Bahr, *Nobody Ever Told Me (or My Mother) That!: Everything from Bottles and Breathing to Healthy Speech Development* (Arlington, TX: Sensory World, 2010); *How to Feed Your Baby and Toddler Right* (Arlington, TX: Future Horizons, 2018).

chian tubes, drain at the back of the throat, roughly where the back of tongue and back of nose meet.[173] The Eustachian tubes share some throat muscles and functions such as swallowing and yawning. Correct swallows promote correct drainage of the fluids from the middle ear. When the drainage is poor the baby or child may develop infections called otitis media, which can be extremely painful. Fluid can also sit in the ear, not causing infection or pain but affecting a baby's hearing, impacting speech and language development. It's not unusual for bottle-fed babies, particularly those who lie down and feed, to develop middle ear fluid and related hearing difficulties.[174]

Being able to hold the jaws closed helps the tongue rest against the upper jaw, also maintaining the upper jaw shape. This is important because the upper jaw forms both the roof of the mouth and the floor of the nose. A poorly shaped upper jaw – too high, too arched or too narrow – leads to dental problems and airway issues common in children with sleep-disordered breathing. A narrow upper jaw is associated with narrow nasal passages. These kids find it hard it to breathe through their nose, and keep their tongue up, and the process reinforces itself. By contrast, developing a healthy, broad upper jaw helps open up the nasal air spaces for nose breathing, mitigating the airway-related sleep disorders commonly related to upper jaw dimension.[175] Developing good body strength and posture is also part of this essential process. Alignment of the head, neck and body makes a big influence on tongue, lip and jaw position. It's like a big body puzzle and all the pieces have to fit together and work together. Tongue up, lips together, back straight.

173 C. Brennan-Jones, R. Eikelboom, A. Jacques, D. Swanepoel, M. Atlas, A. Whitehouse, S. Jamieson and W. Oddy, 'Protective Benefit of Predominant Breastfeeding against Otitis Media May Be Limited to Early Childhood: Results from a Prospective Birth Cohort Study', Clinical Otolaryngology 42, no. 1 (2016), https://doi.org10.1111/coa.12652.

174 Michele Vargas Garcia, Marisa Frasson De Azevedo, José Ricardo Gurgel Testa and Cyntia Barbosa Laureano Luiz, 'The Influence of the Type of Breastfeeding on Middle Ear Conditions in Infants', Brazilian Journal of Otorhinolaryngology 78, no. 1 (2012), https://doi.org/10.1590/s1808-86942012000100002.

175 Christian Guilleminault and Shannon S. Sullivan, 'Towards Restoration of Continuous Nasal Breathing as the Ultimate Treatment Goal in Pediatric Obstructive Sleep Apnea', Enliven: Pediatrics and Neonatal Biology, no. 01 (2014), https://doi.org/10.18650/2379-5824.11001.

Michelle Emanuel recommends more tummy time. She works with babies and has developed the therapeutic TummyTime!™ Method[176] to help babies develop strong posture and alignment.

What can get in the way of ideal postures? When babies are born with a tongue-tie, it can be difficult for the tongue to rest against the roof of the mouth.[177] The piece of connecting tissue under the tongue is called a lingual frenulum, which, when short, is commonly referred to as a tongue-tie. There are degrees of shortness or restriction that are best measured by the effect of tongue-tie on how well the tongue can move or where it can rest comfortably. If tongue mobility is restricted and interfering with breastfeeding or causing a mother discomfort during breastfeeding, then it is usually snipped. Releasing a tongue-tie is so important for babies and mothers that in Brazil, a national law was passed in 2014 requiring all babies to have a tongue-tie inspection at birth. However, it's important to get a thorough assessment to ensure the issue is caused by frenulum restriction and not another functional problem or feeding technique issue. Some oro-motor issues can look like tongue restriction, but a period of therapy can resolve it. A team approach by experienced health professionals is best to determine the problem and the most appropriate treatment, especially considering that some babies' feeding problems can be resolved by specialist support from a lactation nurse.

WHAT YOU CAN DO

After reading this, you'll understand why I promote breastfeeding as the best way to optimise your child's airway health. Unfortunately, bottle-feeding does not achieve the same result. When bottle-feeding, a baby's tongue, cheek and lip muscles function quite differently, requiring much less muscle effort and the baby can still drink and 'fill-up' so there is no red flag to correct their form (as is essential in breast-

176 Michelle Emanuel, 'TummyTime!™ Method', http://www.TummyTimeMethod.com.
177 Christian Guilleminault, Shehlanoor Huseni and Lauren Lo, 'A Frequent Phenotype for Paediatric Sleep Apnoea: Short Lingual Frenulum', *ERJ Open Research* 2, no. 3 (2016), https://doi.org/10.1183/23120541.00043-2016.

feeding). The pressure system that creates milk flow in breastfeeding is non-existent in bottle-feeding. Consequently, bottles encourage incorrect sucking, jaw movement and tongue position. The palate moulds around the bottle (as it does in a thumb-suck or dummy habit) and a high, narrow shape is encouraged, with the tongue sitting low at rest rather than up in the upper jaw, maintaining jaw shape for good airway development. Babies and young children who lie down with a bottle are also at risk of middle ear fluid and infections.[178]

There are many and varied reasons for choosing to bottle feed a baby and, thankfully, we have the option available. The issue is multi-faceted, impacted by society's attitudes, availability of the right support from lactation consultants for breastfeeding mothers, and, of course, family choices or the necessity to return to work while their babies are very young, making breastfeeding difficult to continue. So, there are challenges and complexities in choice of feeding method.

> **If bottle-feeding is inevitable or your choice, there are several things you can do to promote good facial development**

While encouraging you to pursue breastfeeding your child if possible, if bottle feeding is inevitable or your choice, there are several things you can do to promote good facial development. First, it is imperative to feed upright and never lie a baby down with a bottle, as this has a strong connection to middle ear fluid and middle ear infection.[179] Keep bottle-feeds as upright as possible.

Second, use a bottle that requires the muscles of the face, mouth and throat to mimic sucking during breastfeeding as closely as possible.

178 'Ear infections', *Paediatrics & Child Health* 14, no. 7 (2009): 465–66, https://doi.org/10.1093/pch/14.7.465.
179 Garcia et al., 'The Influence of the Type of Breastfeeding on Middle Ear Conditions in Infants'.

Although there is not yet a bottle that can perfectly replicate breast-feeding mechanics, choose a bottle with an adjustable teat that allows adjustment of the flow of milk so that babies are required to suck harder as they get stronger. There are multiple bottle teats developed to mimic the breast, and there is promising research and product development in this area. Check with your local IBCLC (International Board Certified Lactation Consultant) professional who can help mums with these issues.

Third, if your baby is bottle-feeding, supplementing with massage and exercises to encourage use of all the orofacial muscles will be helpful. This will ensure your baby's face, mouth and throat muscles are getting the right kind of activity. You will find some excellent ideas for massage and exercise techniques in Diane Bahr's *Nobody Ever Told Me (or My Mother) That!* and *How to Feed Your Baby and Toddler Right.*

>> Things like raspberries, big noisy kisses, lip pops, ear-to-ear smiles and duck clucks are perfect for this

Whatever feeding technique you are using, engaging in the following games will encourage development of facial and oral muscle control. As soon as your baby can watch and copy you, 'model' faces that encourage your baby's oral and facial muscles to move to their full range of movement. Things like raspberries, big noisy kisses, lip pops, ear-to-ear smiles and duck clucks are perfect for this. Many babies love making noises and love the game of copying mummy or daddy. As soon as you see or hear your baby make any of the faces or sounds, respond with excitement and make lots of eye contact, and they will do it more. Peek-a-boo is a great game for encouraging babies to look intently and laugh a lot. A big, deep laugh is a great workout for the throat and face. Also, use lots of approved 'chew' toys. Encourage your baby to chew, chew, chew.

For good ear drainage, certain activities can help activate the back-of-throat region and the muscles around the ear drainage tubes. The following exercises are suitable for young children (as soon as they can copy) and school kids. They are designed to promote muscle movement in the throat to assist with ear clearing. Some can also help when kids have trouble equalising their ears on plane flights:

- **The big bear yawn:** Imagine you are big, smiley bear just waking from your big winter sleep. Do the biggest ever yawn.

- **Don't catch flies:** Now do the biggest ever yawn and try to keep your lips closed at the same time.

- **Smiley shark:** Open your mouth like a big, happy shark and show me all your teeth, pretending to catch a big load of fish.

- **Silly cow chew:** Pretend you are a cow, chewing on a big mouthful of delicious grass. Let your jaw move side-to-side to crush the grass, and remember to keep your lips shut tight.

- **Deep sea diver:** Pretend you are a diver diving for treasure. As you go down under water, you need to close your nose tight with your fingers, snap your lips shut, puff out your cheeks and blow out, not letting air out of your lips.

- **The happy bulldog:** Smile your biggest smile like a big, happy bulldog, with your lower jaw pushed forward and your lips closed tight.

- **Bunny hop and other bouncy games:** Bounce, bounce and bounce around like a bunny – or bounce, bounce, bounce on a trampoline.

Any middle ear problems that persist should be managed by your GP or your ear, nose and throat doctor.

Nose breathing

Lots of kids these days have a problem with nose breathing. Kids who don't breathe regularly through their noses may have flaccid or swollen lips, an open mouth, inflamed gums, sunken, dark areas under the eyes and slumped shoulders. They chew with their mouths open and often lick their lips because their lips dry out. Many of the younger ones who have this habit drool and have difficulty controlling their saliva. They may end up with a red rash around their mouth and dry, cracked lips.

Mouth breathing is not merely a cosmetic issue. Its dangers are greater than poor oral hygiene or the accompanying bad breath. Mouth breathing has accompanying myofunctional habits (mouth open, tongue low and forward), that lead to non-ideal face and jaw development,[180] rendering children more vulnerable to sleep-disordered breathing.[181,182] To facilitate good facial development, the tongue should rest up fully on the palate, lips should rest together and the back and shoulders should be straight and tall.

When sleeping, mouth breathing is also a problem. Sleeping with your mouth open makes the mouth acidic and dry and therefore prone to tooth decay and bad breath. It leads to non-optimal resting postures of the the tongue and lips during sleep. If a baby or child is mouth breathing and lying on their back, the lower jaw and tongue can lapse back, further narrowing the airway. While mouth breathing is not a severe condition like OSA, it is certainly enough to contribute to sleep fragmentation and disturbed sleep quality.

Mouth breathing can start due to underlying allergies, colds, asthma, nasal obstruction, asymmetrical or narrow nose structure, or having large tonsils and adenoids. Simply, when nasal passages are blocked, it can be difficult to breathe through your nose. The Catch-22 is that the more you mouth breathe, the more mucous is produced, which then

---

180 Meir H. Kryger, Thomas Roth and William C. Dement, *Principles and Practice of Sleep Medicine* (Philadelphia, PA: Elsevier, 2017).

181 Carlos Torre and Christian Guilleminault, 'Establishment of nasal breathing should be the ultimate goal to secure adequate craniofacial and airway development in children', *Jornal de Pediatria*, 2017, https://doi.org/10.1016/j.jped.2017.08.002.

182 Chad M. Ruoff and Christian Guilleminault, 'Orthodontics and sleep-disordered breathing', *Sleep and Breathing* 16, no. 2 (2011), https://doi.org/10.1007/s11325-011-0534-9.

increases congestion.[183] The nose then does not function at its best because it is not being used.

Nose breathing, on the other hand, brings eighteen per cent more oxygen to the brain and promotes full expression of sleep cycles, which helps effective, regenerative sleep. Nose breathing prepares air for the body, encourages adequate saliva production and fresh breath, contributes to optimal palatal development and promotes engagement of the parasympathetic nervous system, the body's calming mechanism, thus reducing stress.[184]

There is also nitric oxide released during nose breathing. This has a natural 'antibiotic' effect and improves uptake of oxygen between the lungs and the brain.

WHAT YOU CAN DO

Encouraging nose breathing in your kids can be a lot of fun, and you can create challenges or games to help build good habits.

The nose is nature's perfect instrument for taking air into the body because it has three engines – a heater to get the air ready for your body, a filter to make sure no sneaky germs get into your body and a humidifier to make sure the air is not too dry for your body. Kids love this concept: 'You have three engines in your nose. Do you know what they are?'

With babies who have a habit of keeping their mouth open, gently and regularly adjust their body, head and neck position and close their lips to encourage nose breathing (as long as they are not congested).

To help kids aged four or older unblock their nose, use the following exercise. Ask the child to breathe in and out of the nose, then hold the

183 Seo-Young Lee, Christian Guilleminault, Hsiao-Yean Chiu, and Shannon S. Sullivan, 'Mouth breathing, 'nasal disuse', and pediatric sleep-disordered breathing', Sleep and Breathing 19, no. 4 (2015), https://doi.org/10.1007/s11325-015-1154-6.

184 Ornish Living, 'Breathe Your Way Into Balance', Huffpost, 2017, https://www.huffingtonpost.com/ornish-living/breathe-your-way-into-bal_b_7285090.html.

nose and sway until a breath is needed. Once a breath is needed, the nostrils are released, letting all the air slowly into the nose. I usually get kids to hold something between their lips, like a tongue depressor or ice cream stick, to help them remember to take their breath through the

nose. You can call their attention to this by saying, 'Did your mouth try and take the air before your nose? Let's try again and see if your nose can take in the air this time.'

You can also challenge kids to breathe so quietly you can't even hear their breathing. You can up the stakes: 'I bet your dad can't do this'; 'I bet your mum can't'; 'See if your mum can remember to breathe through her nose'; 'Let's see who can breathe so quietly no one can hear'; 'Let's see who can breathe in and out of the nose and keep their whole body still.'

Kids love this stuff. Some may giggle a lot, and it takes some skill to hold something in their lips while they're giggling *and* breathing through their nose. If your child is giggling and still holding their lips tightly closed, though, they are most likely working their back-of-throat muscles very well, which is great!

A great resource for teaching healthy breathing is the Buteyko method, a breathing technique created by a Ukrainian born doctor, Konstantin Buteyko to help treat asthma and other respiratory conditions. The crux of the method is to eliminate the habit of 'over-breathing', which develops with mouth breathers and other medical conditions. More information about this method can be found at: http://buteykoclinic.com/buteykochildren.

>> healthy development of the airway (and therefore, healthy sleep) goes hand in hand with using the muscles correctly. Chewing is key to this development

Moving to solid food

As I've discussed throughout this chapter, healthy development of the airway (and therefore, healthy sleep) goes hand in hand with using the muscles correctly. Chewing is key to this development.[185]

When babies chew, it stimulates bone growth of the jaws and face. Great chewing, sucking and swallowing create movement of muscles against the bone to which they are connected, influencing almost every bone in the face and skull. That movement then stimulates growth.[186] In the same way as exercise is recommended for people recovering from bone breaks or those with osteoporosis, chewing influences the bone health of the jaws, face and skull. Chewing is also essential for brain development and function as well as for concentration and calming stress.[187,188] Science has also found that good chewing is essential for digestion and preparing food for breakdown in your stomach. In later life, effective chewing can facilitate general health and wellbeing.[189]

Poor chewing is associated with narrow upper jaw structure. We are usually not aware of how much is going on in our mouth when we bite, chew and swallow. Biting happens at the front teeth, then the tongue is

185 Licia Coceani Paskay, 'Chewing, Biting, Clenching, Bruxing And Oral Health', Oral Health Group, 2018, https://www.oralhealthgroup.com/features/1003919890.
186 Daniel Lieberman, *Evolution of the Human Head*, (Harvard University Press, 2011)
187 Sandrine Thuret, 'You Can Grow New Brain Cells. Here's How', *Ted.com*, recorded June, 2015, https://www.ted.com/talks/sandrine_thuret_you_can_grow_new_brain_cells_here_s_how.
188 Yoshiyuki Hirano and Minoru Onozuka, 'Chewing and Attention: A Positive Effect on Sustained Attention', *BioMed Research International* 2015 (2015), https://doi.org/10.1155/2015/367026.
189 Akinori Tasaka, Manaki Kikuchi, Kousuke Nakanishi, Takayuki Ueda, Shuichiro Yamashita, and Kaoru Sakurai, 'Psychological stress-relieving effects of chewing - Relationship between masticatory function-related factors and stress-relieving effects', *Journal of Prosthodontic Research* 62, no. 1 (2018), https://doi.org/10.1016/j.jpor.2017.05.003.

busily moving the food between our back teeth, positioning it for chewing and then for swallowing near the back of the tongue. The sides of the tongue are deftly positioning food on the centre of the tongue ready for a swallow. To swallow, food is positioned on the back third of the tongue and propelled backwards in a wave-like motion against the hard palate. When the food hits around about the tonsil area, a swallow reflex is triggered, and the throat muscles take over after that to deliver the food further down to the stomach. It is no wonder kids with big tonsils shy away from textured foods and can only cope with small amounts food – there's not a lot of room back there and swallowing can hurt!

The chewing motion in babies starts very early, usually by six months, and typically matures by twelve months, and by this time the tongue tip should be able to elevate up to the gum pad just behind the top teeth for a mature swallow. This tongue tip placement for a mature swallow is the same as for speech sounds 't', 'd', 'n' and 'l'. Meanwhile, teeth are needed to clear food from the lips, a movement that is the same position as what we use for 'f' and 'v' sounds. By the age of two, littlies should be able to chew and swallow perfectly, although vigilance is still required when kids are chewing their way through a plate of food, as the most common cause of non-fatal choking in young children is food.[190]

>> many children are not learning the skill of chewing early enough, due to the common use of bottles, sippy-cups and soft foods

The problem is that many children are not learning the skill of chewing early enough and they develop a kind of learned helplessness. This is partly due to the common use of bottles, sippy-cups and soft foods. Unfortunately, today we often introduce textured foods into our children's diets too late, focusing on soft food. Soft foods require no muscle work and are linked to

190 'Choking Prevention For Children', Health.Ny.Gov, 2018, https://www.health.ny.gov/prevention/injury_prevention/choking_prevention_for_children.htm.

modification of whole facial structure,[191] with soft diets leading to small, recessed lower jaws, crooked teeth and a compromised upper airway.

Starting to chew late by-passes early developmental opportunities. Some common chewing problems or habits include: one sided chewing and gulping food down before it has been chewed properly. Mouth breathing disrupts chewing efficiency.[192] Poor chewing is asymmetrical, open-mouthed, too fast or too slow, noisy or incomplete, meaning that food may be swallowed in chunks and not fully prepared for the digestion process in the stomach, leading to digestive issues like bloating. Most kids I meet in clinic are chewing exactly like this when I first meet them – even school age kids, teenagers and some adults.

>> the most compelling reason to chew well is facilitation of healthy orofacial development and a healthy airway

Many parents I see in the clinic are unaware of the way their kids are chewing as their focus is primarily on manners. Manners have their place, but by far, the most compelling reason to chew well is facilitation of healthy orofacial development and a healthy airway. The way the muscles are used and how well the food is chewed will achieve success in both manners and good chewing.

WHAT YOU CAN DO

You can do a lot to help your child develop healthy chewing habits.

For babies, be sure to introduce appropriate food textures at the right times. Babies usually start being spoon fed solid foods at around six months old. To spoon-feed effectively, a baby needs to watch you eat from a spoon. Make sure they are sitting straight upright and well

191 Sheldon et al., *Principles and Practice of Pediatric Sleep Medicine*. 275–80.
192 Miho Nagaiwa, Kaori Gunjigake and Kazunori Yamaguchi, 'The Effect of Mouth Breathing on Chewing Efficiency', *The Angle Orthodontist* 86, no. 2 (2016), https://doi.org/10.2319/020115-80.1.

supported, wait for them to open their mouth for the food, close their lips on a flat-bowl spoon (choosing the right size for your baby's mouth is key) then withdraw the spoon in a rhythmical fashion, making sure to keep it level – and try not to scrape up. By the time a baby is two years old, they should be able to feed themselves just like we do. Always re-member – posture, posture, posture. Sitting upright with the chin in a neutral position (not up, not down) is an important part of chewing well. It really helps if they are at your eye level so when they are looking at you, their natural head position is neutral.

Seventy-five per cent of food should be chewy or crunchy. If you can achieve this as early as possible, you have a great start to myo-opti-misation. So, while most people start their baby on soft rice cereal, minimise it and offer finger food. Finger food allows a baby to explore texture, self-feed and develop the oro-motor control required to handle textured food safely. Let your baby choose from a range of solid foods that require biting, gnawing and chewing,[193] but stay present for when your baby needs extra help or caution is required.[194]

>> Chewing starts even before the teeth come in. In fact, chewing can *help* the teeth come in!

Chewing starts even before the teeth come in (usually between five and nine months). In fact, chewing can *help* the teeth come in! Encourag-ing your baby to chew on non-food items (such as the side of your finger pad) can start much younger if your baby needs some jaw develop-ment and oral coordination to help with their breathing, sucking and swallowing. Baby-safe feeders (mesh feeders with a cover) can be helpful when introducing your baby to solid foods like chunks of fruit, vegetables or meat. They are particularly helpful for kids with compromised oro-motor control like low muscle

193 Gill Rapley and Tracey Murkett, *Baby-Led Weaning: Helping Your Baby to Love Good Food* (Chatham, Me.: Vermilion, 2008).

194 Nimali Fernando and Melanie Potock, *Parenting in the Kitchen: How to Raise Happy and Healthy Eaters at Every Step in Your Child's Development* (New York, NY: The Experiment, LLC, 2015).

tone or poor sensation in the mouth, or at times you are not able to fully supervise young children.[195]

Many parents are also surprised to learn that children can start drinking from an open cup at six months old. Have babies practise with a little water in cups so if they spill it it's not a big deal. If spillage is an issue, choose a recessed-lidded cup rather than a sippy-cup, as sippy-cups promote the same poor muscle usage as a baby bottle. Additionally, if the spout sits between the teeth, there is a higher chance it will disrupt dental development, like dummy and thumb sucking habits. Spillage seems to be the primary reason parents use sippy-cups, but this isn't an issue with recessed lids as the liquid sits in the rim and doesn't spill. Kids can also use shortened straws that go just past the lips, but not into the mouth.

There are also special, safety-approved sensory toys to assist with chewing and biting. These must be right shape, size and texture for your baby or child's age. In my clinic, I use a range of chewing appliances including Myo Munchees (https://myomunchee.com) whenever I think children (from eighteen months old) need some extra help developing their 'chew' muscles. Kids love to chew, bite and mouth new objects – a stage that can last up to their preschool years and sometimes later.

There are many things you can do to help older kids chew food well. First, make sure your child can comfortably breathe through their nose. Once kids can nose breathe effectively, then it's a matter of chewing the right way. Correct chewing means keeping lips together and engaging both sides of the mouth simultaneously and symmetrically, at a moderate pace and with a mix of vertical and *mini* horizontal jaw movements, until the food is soft and mushy, ready for the stomach.

195 Nancy Ripton and Melanie Potock, *Baby Self-Feeding: Solid Food Solutions to Create Lifelong, Healthy Eating Habits* (Beverly, MA: Fair Winds, 2016).

Once kids know how to chew the right way, you want to establish the habit of good chewing. This takes practice, encouragement and good modelling. So, at the dinner table you can make a game of chewing well. Here are some ideas to get started (these ideas work mostly with kids after age three or four):

- **Associations:** Associations can help trigger the brain to remember things. This is very helpful when learning behaviour we do not normally think about. For instance, you could talk about how animals chew. Look at dogs, cats, bunnies and giraffes chewing. Pretend you are a giraffe chewing (doing all the wrong things). There are many ways to teach your kids how to chew correctly: 'pompous chew', 'princess chew' or 'chewing with the queen'. I have developed these techniques and used them for more than a decade and they never cease to engage a giggle or two and develop great chewing habits. Pompous chewing engages the top lip to stabilise the jaw, and keep the lips together, rather than the common disorganised jaw movement (which I call 'jazz dancing jaw') that is commonly seen. To start learning how to chew well, stretch your top lip down rhythmically and repeatedly as the teeth open and close for munching, crunching and gnashing food. For a great animal chewing model, the humble capybara is the winner; not perfect but pretty good!

- **Modelling:** When you model good chewing, your children are likely to copy without you ever needing to teach them. By doing this they will know exactly how to do their 'pompous' chewing.

- **Rewards:** Be lavish with your praise when kids try hard and do well with chewing. 'Wow, I just saw you doing perfect pompous chewing!' Joining in and interacting with them is great encouragement to keep little people doing well. You can set challenges e.g. how many times can you chew one mouthful in 30 seconds? Keep it light-hearted and fun. If it gets too didactic, they won't enjoy it at all.

- **Visual reminders:** Put up photos or pictures of pompous chewing at or near the table, so every time you child sees the photo they remember how they are supposed to chew. For example, you could make a laminated placemat with special pictures of a pompous face or capybara coloured by your child. The brain adapts quickly to visual reminders – reminders often stop working within two weeks – so it is important to change images as soon as they lose their potency.

- **Fun with food:** Something we do regularly in the clinic, which kids absolutely love, is to get creative with food. We lay out a range of food choices and a picture of something we want them to make with the food, such as a ship or an underwater scene or a funny face. While making the food, we identify the foods by texture – which ones are soft, chewy or crunchy. After making the food, we then systematically eat it, using perfect pompous chewing and smiley swallowing.

- **Music:** Kids really enjoy rhythmic music and songs that roughly follow the same bite/chomp rate as chewing, so why not chew to music? We do it regularly in the clinic with our creative food projects, and it's easy to do at home.

- **My mouth talks to my tummy:** Kids love to know that when they chew well, their mouth and their tummy are having a conversation! When kids understand why they are doing something, they will do it more.

- **Invisible swallowing:** Of course, after chewing comes swallowing, and we need to make sure it's correct. Great swallowing is invisible and silent with no lip bracing or head–body movement: up straight, gentle lip seal, tongue anchoring up against the palate, no noise and no forward tongue movement. If this is not happening, myo-correct is needed (see Chapter 6).

> **>> keep your eyes on the prize – a well-developed facial structure and a healthy airway that will maximise your child's potential for restful, restorative sleep**

There are plenty of ways to encourage the automation of these skills so that they become habit, but family involvement and encouragement is key. In all this, the nutritious quality of food choices is also an essential. As you work on these chewing habits, keep your eyes on the prize – a well-developed facial structure and a healthy airway that will maximise your child's potential for restful, restorative sleep.

For even more great information on the importance of chewing and nutrition and its links to health, I recommend checking out Dr Steven Lin's great book, The Dental Diet: The Surprising Link Between Your Teeth, Real Food, and Life-Changing Natural Health.[196]

Learning to speak well

The muscles used for breathing, sucking, chewing and swallowing are the same muscle systems that work for speech, although the mechanisms for all of these functions are not as simple as 'move muscle A to position B'. There are more complex brain processes that govern speech, not to mention the interplay between speech and language. However, atypical speech habits may develop in conjunction with myofunctional disorders,[197] and it makes sense, given the anatomy and function of the face and mouth.

---

196 Lin, *The Dental Diet*.

197 Robyn Merkel-Walsh, 'AAPPSPA Position Statement - Oral-Motor Therapy', *Talktools*, December 2, 2015, https://talktools.com/blogs/from-the-experts/aappspa-position-statement-oral-motor-therapy.

Most babies start vocalising from two to three months old. Broadly speaking, children start using single words around twelve months of age, then start stringing two words together into an ever-increasing vocabulary by age two.

However, many kids' speech is delayed because they are not receiving the right kind of early stimulation. Many parents don't know how to talk to their baby, and there is a school of thought that you should speak to your baby in 'adult' speak from the beginning to avoid baby talk. It's true that kids do need adult models of language, but they also need exposure to baby talk, toddler talk, lots of singing and everything in between.

Development of intelligible speech sounds into words and sentences is essential to clear communication. The ability to produce clear speech sounds is connected to use of the muscles of the face mouth throat and larynx. Babies imitate facial movement very early,[198] so the sooner your baby starts imitating sounds and copying your exaggerated faces and voices, the sooner and more fully they are activating the upper airway muscle systems, contributing to both upper airway health and communication development. Let's face it, there's nothing like a good belly laugh for opening up the throat muscles. In Chapter 2, I mentioned the Kalahari Bushmen, who have broad jaw structures encouraged by their click language. Many kids I see in clinic cannot elevate the tongue to the roof of the mouth, nor can they make a nice loud sharp click or cluck sound. Yet tongue elevation is critical. Remember the Kalahari bush kids with beautiful, broad, well-developed palates? Our kids need that too.

WHAT YOU CAN DO

To get kids' speech and language off to a great start, it's best to combine activities that are concurrently developing both speech and language skills. Read, talk, hum and sing to your baby while in utero and from the

---

198 Diane Bahr, *Nobody Ever Told Me (or My Mother) That! Everything from Bottles and Breathing to Healthy Speech Development* (Arlington, TX: Sensory World, 2010).

day they are born. While they may not be talking yet, they are certainly listening, and the brain is at the height of its ability to listen, encode sounds and lay down a template for speech and language.[199] Listening is the start of talking, so talk a lot, read a lot and sing a lot. Have fun with words.

>> have fun – encourage your child to do lots of clicks, clucks and smiles

There's a lot more to it than simply mimicking sounds, though. Speech and language development is highly interactive and very much a two-way process.[200] So, when your baby starts sound play, cooing and gurgling, coo and gurgle back because it encourages more of the same – a real two-way interaction. Babies love making all sorts of sounds. They find many new sounds in their own sound play. As soon as you hear it, make a fuss, imitate it, have fun – encourage your child to do lots of clicks, clucks and smiles. This early sound imitation will not only help develop speech, oro-facial muscle control, and verbal skills, but it will also create a sense of fun and connection and 'conversation' between the two of you. It is also very important to eliminate or limit dummy use; when there's a dummy or thumb or fingers in the mouth, not much sound play can happen.

As your baby starts to make a wider range of sounds, mimic them and add more vocal intonation into your own speaking (so make your speaking voice musical and interesting). Babies love to hear the music of voice. Whenever your baby vocalises or 'talks', vocalise and talk back to them. Get in the habit of explaining the world around you, in adult speak, but also add in elements of dramatisation and exaggeration – be silly and make lots of faces that your baby will start to follow.

199   Patricia K. Kuhl, 'Brain Mechanisms in Early Language Acquisition', *Neuron* 67, no. 5 (2010), https://doi.org/10.1016/j.neuron.2010.08.038.

200   Bjorn Carey, 'Talking Directly to Toddlers Strengthens Their Language Skills, Stanford Research Shows', *Stanford University*, October 15, 2013, https://news.stanford.edu/news/2013/october/fernald-vocab-development-101513.html.

Humming, singing, talking, laughing and clucking all activate the muscles of the mouth, face and throat, as do speech, voice, facial expression, chewing, sucking and swallowing. They all contribute to developing a healthy upper airway.

There are many good resources online that can help you develop your child's speech. The Speech Pathology Australia website (www.speechpathologyaustralia.org.au) and the American Speech-Language-Hearing Association website (www.asha.org) both are a good starting point. I also like the Hanen approach to teaching language. You can learn more about Hanen at www.hanen.org/Programs/For-Parents/It-Takes-Two-to-Talk.

Games and activities that promote an open airway

Kids have a lot of fun making sounds and pulling faces, which is terrific, as these activities are so helpful for upper airway development. In the same way you may take your child to the park to play, have fresh air and get strong, face and mouth 'gym' can optimise the muscles, help kids be more aware of the muscles and develop control. Remember, these activities are for kids who do not have a diagnosed problem. If your child is in therapy, this approach can supplement traditional speech, sound or phonological therapy, especially when where your child is not progressing, and it is great for kids with low muscle tone.

If you want to do some extra activities that are fun, try some of the following resistance exercises, which we use in my clinic to promote movement and action at the back of the throat:

- **Cheek balloons:** Fill up your cheeks with air, then try to hold the air as someone pops them. You can also do this activity with water, make a water pump.

- **Cheek pokes:** Push your tongue into your cheek while someone pushes against your tongue from outside the cheek.

- **Suck thick liquids:** Try drinking a thick smoothie with a wide straw.

- **Blow bubbles into thick liquids:** Try blowing bubbles into a thick smoothie with a wide straw.

- **Blow up balloons:** Use a one-way valve to help blow up a balloon, or blow up a balloon and seal the opening with your lips in between blows. Make sure it's a nose breath then a blow

- **Play wind instruments:** Play, play, play, making sure your child is taking a breath in through the nose in between each blow.

- **Try 'Lady and the Tramp' pasta noodle scoop:** Remember the Disney movie scene where the romancing dogs scoop the noodle with their lips and end up kissing? This can be done with al dente pasta noodle, long peel from apples or carrots or any other long, stringy food. (Original exercise created by speech language pathologist Dan Garliner.)[201]

In the clinic, I always talk about 'chipping away, a little everyday to build new habits.' Families manage best with all these suggestions and activities when they are integrated into what you do daily anyway: bath times, meal times, play times or car trips. With myo-optimise, there is so much you can do with your children as part of everyday life. However, if you want assistance, find an experienced myofunctional practitioner close by and they will help you by providing guidance, accountability and lots of strategies to get myo-optimise working for your family.

The impacts of this therapy on a child's everyday life and development are phenomenal. In fact, parents can benefit too. Recently one parent who had their child in clinic and did all the exercises with her little one stopped snoring! When working with kids in the clinic, I discover that many parents have poor myofunctional habits that they become aware of during our sessions and they benefit from doing the training too, starting with foundation exercises until the patterns become completely automatic.

201 Daniel Garliner, *Myofunctional Therapy* (Philadelphia: W.B. Saunders, 1981).

Encouraging the muscles to rest in the right place

So often we see kids (and older people) sitting with their mouths open, tongues low or forward and slumpy postures. None of this is ideal. What are the ideal postures? We have seen before that ideal position is tongue resting fully in the upper jaw with lips gently resting together and a straight back. Keeping lips together ensures that nose breathing is happening, while a straight back ensures that the airway is in its ideal position. It's the magic three postures.

Here is the graphic representation I have been using for the last ten years.

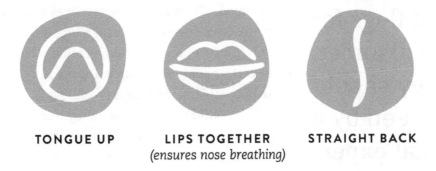

TONGUE UP   **LIPS TOGETHER**   **STRAIGHT BACK**
                       (ensures nose breathing)

Because kids learn much better by associations than by mechanical instructions, I developed a mantra for them from this set of instructions:

- Tongue up on the roof of the mouth,
- Lips gently resting together, and
- Back straight.

Just saying the word 'mantra' reminds them to instantly move into perfect postures. Say 'mantra' to any of the kids that work with me and see what happens. Boom, straight into position. I am constantly amazed at how quickly kids adopt this mantra and have fun with it. We practise it in many different ways, and families are shown how they can assimilate it into family life over time until it becomes a habit.

It is just as important to have the muscles resting in the right place when they have nothing else to do as it is to have them moving correctly when they have something to do.

When to bring in the experts

If your child's sleep problems and symptoms of SDB are mild, then all the information on environment, routine and myo will be invaluable for you.

>> If your child is exhibiting any red flags for a sleep disorder, they should be seen by a medical expert

If your child is older and has some deeply ingrained poor habits, don't be disheartened – it is never too late to change. Life events and difficulties happen. The way we live our lives is rarely textbook, and there is no such thing as a perfect life, perfect parent or perfect child. The key is to start as soon as possible. Once you realise there is a problem, take steps to address it. If you think your child has developed a myofunctional disorder, then it's time to see a myofunctional practitioner for myo-correction.

As a lifeguard of your child's sleep, perhaps you have found your child metaphorically drowning or struggling. You may know within yourself that expert assistance is required. If your child is exhibiting any red flags for a sleep disorder, they should be seen by a medical expert. You'll need to seek out the medical, dental and allied health practitioners who have a special interest in sleep disorders and upper airway health. In the following chapter, I'll share how you can approach your search for the right practitioners to help your child sleep. In your role as lifeguard, it's time to call the expert team.

CHAPTER SIX

Should we work with a specialist?

At eight years old, Jillian was a bundle of energy. She would wriggle and squirm constantly, so much so that her nickname was 'Wriggle Jiggle'. Her parents assumed it was just the way she was. She had never slept through a full night due to nightmares. Instead, she would wake terrified and unable to go back to sleep most nights, and the whole family's sleep was disrupted by her night-time shenanigans. During the day, Jillian's anxiety was easily triggered by hints and suggestions of scary things, which would then feature in her nightmares. She was unable to sit still during the day and fidgeted constantly. Jillian was wired.

Jillian was referred to me by a local dentist for speech issues (lisp) and thumb sucking. When I met Jillian at first assessment we found a range of red flags. She was still sucking her thumb at eight years old and had a significant myofunctional disorder. Dental and structural assessment showed an anterior open bite (upper and lower front teeth do not meet) and a crossbite (the upper jaw is narrower than the lower jaw) with a high, narrow, arched upper jaw and a recessed lower jaw and tooth agenesis (Jillian had four teeth missing) – all red flags for small jaw development and airway issues. While there was no suggestion of ADHD, her constant movement suggested the relentless activity typically associated with sleep deprivation and poor sleep quality.[202]

Because of Jillian's thumb sucking and the size, shape and position of her jaws, the muscles in her mouth, face and throat had maladapted.

---

202 Dana C. Won, Christian Guilleminault, Peter J. Koltai, Stacey D. Quo, Martin T. Stein and Irene M. Loe, 'It Is Just Attention-Deficit Hyperactivity Disorder … or Is It?' *Journal of Developmental & Behavioral Pediatrics*, 2017, https://doi.org/10.1097/dbp.0000000000000386.

Her tongue's resting position was forward instead of up, and her chin was overworking when her lips were together. All of these red flags suggested airway restriction and possible SDB, which could lie beneath her light sleep, disrupted sleep patterns and nightmares. Jillian's mum described anxiety around her sleep pattern. Surprisingly, there were no reports from the school about social, academic or behavioural issues.

At that point, my interpretation of symptoms was based on supposition only, and we needed to get Jillian a diagnosis by a medical and dental specialist. But it helped to come up with a plan of action. When discussing courses of action, Jillian's parents were encouraged to see a sleep specialist, but at the time they only considered an orthodontic consultation, which they pursued to explore possible links to jaw development, sleep fragmentation and airway, based on a number of relevant research papers they had read.

Jillian had a thumb sucking habit and was diagnosed with a moderate myofunctional disorder related to structural anomalies, including high narrow palate. She was on 'nocturnal airway watch', given the severity of her sleep profile. After six months of 'airway-centric' dental treatment, which opened her airway and corrected her crossbite, alongside our myo-correct program for her thumb-sucking habit, Jillian started sleeping through the night. In fact, for the first time in eight years, Jillian slept through the night for three nights in a row. In those three days, she was like a new child – her intense night-time fear diminished and she was able to sit still and focus during the day. Wriggle Jiggle was now Mademoiselle Zen. Jillian's mum was pleased that the better sleep had not quelled her delightful personality in the least.

>> for the first time in eight years, Jillian slept through the night for three nights in a row

After Jillian's dental and orthodontic treatment was complete, we resumed myofunctional therapy to ensure that her myo-habits would fully stabilise, support the upper jaw changes and stimulate growth for the

>> **Jillian's parents had tried a lot of things to improve Jillian's sleep habits, including the 'musical beds' approach, but it had not solved the issues**

lower jaw through chewing and swallowing exercises. I noticed how much calmer she was and how she was able to sit still in our sessions. By the time we finished the last session, Jillian's mum reported that she was sleeping through the night without waking regularly now, and the whole family was getting a good night's sleep.

Jillian's parents had tried a lot of things to improve Jillian's sleep habits, including the 'musical beds' approach, but it had not solved the issues. They eventually tried a reward system to entice her out of her bedtime stalling tactics; however, this was after the dental intervention. It proved useful for breaking her delay tactics habit. By all accounts, changing undesirable 'sleep hygiene' behaviours for Jillian was a step-by-step process and is a work in progress. At each step we checked back in to measure progress and changes.

While there is a lot you can do on your own to improve your child's sleep, especially when it comes to their behaviour, routine and environment, the benefit of getting expert help is that you may find a faster solution to a treatable problem. Jillian is a great example of this. Experienced practitioners have seen thousands of kids with problems like yours. They have worked in hospitals where they have seen the worst possible cases and the best possible outcomes as well as very mild cases that can be solved with subtle tweaks and changes that make a big difference.

With expert help from sleep and airway-focused professionals, you will also benefit from an official diagnosis, access to the most up-to-date research and methods, the best treatment options, support on the journey, clear and realistic expectations about your child's improvement (and milestones along the way) and the depth of expertise that comes with a coordinated team approach. The ultimate goal is to solve the problem and help your child sleep well.

In this chapter, I'll share a list of the different specialists you might like to consider and how to choose the right fit for your child and your family.

Who can help with sleep disorders?

There are many different specialists and health practitioners who may be able to help as part of your child's sleep and airway team. For most children a team will be required to ensure a complete treatment approach. Keep in mind that the primary and adjunctive team will vary according to your child's problem and a sleep specialist is usually the team lead. The team may consist of two, three or multiple specialists, depending on your child's needs, and those needs may change over time. You may be working with one team member as a priority for a period of time, but as treatment priorities change so will the area of expertise. Remember, the treatment for influencing growth of the airway is short with ninety per cent growth complete before a child hits puberty.

Here's an overview of the medical and dental specialists who may assist with disordered sleep and sleep disorders. I have also outlined a range of allied health professionals who have sleep and airway symptoms on their radar, as they may become important members of your 'dream team'.

GENERAL MEDICAL PRACTITIONER (GP)

The family doctor is often the first place a mum or dad will ask for help when they know there are issues. GPs have a critical role to play in identifying the early signs of upper airway problems. They may be the first to identify the need for ENT, sleep physician, feeding specialist, speech pathologist or myofunctional practitioner. They are also likely to flag hallmarks of ADHD and any child who requires screening for a sleep disorder.

>> There are three top questions for parents: Are my children getting enough sleep? Are they waking refreshed? Are they getting good quality sleep? Any 'no' is a red flag

By intervening early, GPs can help everybody. But, given that sleep medicine is still an emerging field of medicine, sleep and airway related disorders are not always top of every GP's radar. While there are many GPs who are quick to recognise and refer for sleep problems, many have a 'wait and see' approach. But how long do you want to wait?

This is why it's important for parents to be aware of red flags that can lead to abnormal breathing, including all conditions from Chapter 2 (See page 81). As a proactive parent, you can then discuss any red flags you want investigated further and request that your GP help you with a referral to the right specialist.

Along with the GP, early childhood nurses have contact with all preschool children at regular health checks. They are in the prime position to screen a child's 'sleep formula' from the very first visit, checking whether they're getting the right amount of sleep and good sleep quality. They may only need to ask two simple questions: 'Is the child getting enough sleep for their age?' and 'Does the child wake well rested?'

PAEDIATRICIAN

Paediatricians are concerned with the health of infants, children and teenagers. They provide physical, mental and emotional care for their patients and also treat children suffering from injuries, acute and chronic health problems, and physiological and psychological growth and developmental concerns. Like GPs, they are in the front line with a large population of children and have a critical role to play in flagging sleep problems and airway symptoms. They will be able to help with any underlying diagnosis of conditions that raise red flags for sleep and airway related sleep disorders. Again, you can request their help to investigate sleep and airway health.

A paediatrician may be the first specialist to see a child with behavioural and developmental disturbances associated with sleep disorders. Some kids are born with conditions that increase their risk of SDB, and the child's care will depend on their paediatrician's diagnosis, as parents often prioritise a paediatrician's advice over all others.

For instance, a paediatrician may be the first one to see an infant struggling with breastfeeding and be able to identify traits like low muscle tone or tongue-tie restrictions affecting feeding. This would ideally result in the paediatrician referring patients on to a certified lactation consultant for good breastfeeding support or a myofunctional practitioner to develop orofacial muscle function. However, these ideas may not be fully on your paediatrician's radar because the field of sleep medicine is still relatively young and orofacial myofunctional science is an emerging discipline.

As Dr. Judy Owens suggests, 'All children presenting for evaluation of psychiatric and neurodevelopmental disorders should routinely be assessed for insomnia and sleep disorders.'[203] As the field of precision medicine evolves, the earliest signs of airway related sleep disorders will take more prominence in medical investigations. Once again, as a parent you can start a discussion about the red flags with your child's paediatrician or request a referral.

SLEEP PHYSICIAN OR PAEDIATRIC SLEEP SPECIALIST

A sleep physician or specialist will decide if your child needs a sleep study (polysomnography or PSG). They will also do other investigations like a physical exam and blood test. They may suggest actigraphy, a monitoring system that tracks and measures your child's rest and sleep cycles over the period of a week.

203 Owens, 'Comorbidity of Insomnia'.

>> A sleep study is the current definitive test for sleep disorder

A sleep study, which is the current definitive test for sleep disorder, is an overnight sleep test. A small plastic tube is placed under the nose to measure airflow, two elastic straps are put around the chest and stomach to measure breathing, a probe is put on the finger to measure oxygen, a sensor is put on the skin to measure carbon dioxide and another plastic sensor is placed above the top lip to measure breathing through the mouth. All the sensors are then connected to a computer, which monitors the study and produces graphs that show what's happening during sleep. Kids' clinics are set up to be kid friendly spaces; Dr Papadopoulos for example, has Sully from *Monsters, Inc.* as a regular feature.[204] Each child stays overnight with a parent.

Why would a parent want a sleep study or further evaluation for their child? While screening questionnaires are very helpful, they are not diagnostic and simply identify the need for further assessment. A sleep study provides that assessment. Anyone whose kids have serious sleep red flags should consider seeing a sleep specialist to determine what's going on. Certain red flags are redder than others; if your child gasps, chokes or snores heavily, these need to be medically investigated.

There are some drawbacks to sleep studies. Because a PSG is not undertaken at home, it can be challenging for children (and parents), and it's difficult to ensure accurate testing because kids move a lot. They are expensive and not scalable; in other words, we have way more kids who need the tests than there is capacity to test them. Specialists are working very hard to come up with an accurate home testing format, which would make testing more easily available to more families and decrease the stress and financial burden on both the family and the health care system.[205] Experts have been working on alternatives to PSG for some time now. Dr Colin Sullivan, inventor of CPAP, has developed a promis-

---

204 'Paediatric Sleep Medicine and ENT at St George Private Hospital', video published July 28, 2016, https://www.youtube.com/watch?v=-U0dBOLLQ8c.

205 Gozal, 'Pediatric Sleep Apnea: Clinical and Diagnostic Aspects'.

ing home test sleep mat called Sonomat. 'The Sonomat accurately diagnoses SDB in children using current metrics. In addition, it permits quantification of partial airway obstruction that can be used to better describe paediatric SDB. Its non-contact design makes it ideal for use with children.[206] Other home sleep tests are in development and clinical trials, such as Esprit Nova, aim to provide accurate home testing and drastically reduce waiting times and cost of accurate testing.

That said, PSGs are currently the gold standard method for accurately determining what is happening during sleep. Accurate testing is invaluable, and the results are then used to determine treatment.

After thorough examination, if your child is diagnosed with a sleep disorder or disordered sleep, your sleep specialist will recommend a suitable treatment for your child. They may give advice on whether CPAP, medications or nutritional supplements are required. They may advise on sleep position and many other aspects of sleep hygiene or refer you to another health practitioner, like a psychologist, to assist with behaviours or routines. If surgery is necessary, they may refer you to the relevant medical specialist, or if they think palatal expansion will be helpful, they may refer you to a dentist or orthodontist. They may refer you to other medical specialists: ENT, endocrinology or genetics. There are many specialists that may contribute to management of a sleep disorder with underlying medical condition.

DENTAL SPECIALIST

Paediatric dentists are dedicated to children's oral health from infancy through the teen years. They have the experience and qualifications to care for a child's teeth, gums and mouth throughout the various stages of childhood.

---

206 Mark B. Norman, Sonia M. Pithers, Arthur Y. Teng and Karen A. Waters, 'Validation of the Sonomat Against PSG and Quantitative Measurement of Partial Upper Airway Obstruction in Children With Sleep-Disordered Breathing', *Sleep* 40, no. 3 (2017), https://doi.org/10.1093/sleep/ zsx017.

Ideally, a dentist would be involved in screening for baby's dental and oral care even before the teeth come in. Most parents don't think of having an early oral health screening for their children, and most parents I meet have not had their child's first dental check-up by the time the child starts preschool.

Some dentists are proactive in the identification and treatment of airway, advocating for the early correction of oral habits and early expansion when a child's jaw growth is off track, discrepant or compromised. Given the mouth, jaws and teeth are the portal to the airway and a significant part of the airway complex, Dr Felix Liao in Virginia, US, talks about the concept of a 'mouth doctor' rather than a 'straight tooth doctor'.[207]

>> Dentists can identify red flags in growth of the mouth and face and any compromise this may place on the airway, along with airway screening for symptoms of SDB or OSA

Dentists can identify red flags in growth of the mouth and face and any compromise this may place on the airway, along with airway screening for symptoms of SDB or OSA. They have measurement tools at their disposal, and while not everyone uses imaging to determine airway volume, there are measurement systems to determine jaw width and height to see if airway growth is on track or not.[208,209] This may include traits and growth patterns that are not associated with a syndrome or other medical condition but will nevertheless impact the airway. Many doctors are reticent to use X-rays for

207 Felix Liao, *Six-Foot Tiger, Three-Foot Cage: Take Charge of Your Health* (Carlsburg, CA: Crescendo Publishing, 2017).

208 Shirley Leibovitz, Yaron Haviv, Yair Sharav, Galit Almoznino, Doron Aframian and Uri Zilberman, 'Pediatric Sleep-Disordered Breathing: Role of the Dentist', *Quintessence Int* 48, no. 8 (2017), https://doi.org/10.3290/j.qi.a38554.

209 Chad M. Ruoff and Christian Guilleminault, 'Orthodontics and Sleep-Disordered Breathing', *Sleep and Breathing* 16, no. 2 (2011), https://doi.org/10.1007/s11325-011-0534-9.

imaging the airway, because of the radiation. CBCT (lower radiation 3D scans) is an alternative, but it's not available in every dental practice.

Your dentist will also look for red flags relating to bad bite (malocclusion): crossbite, high-arched maxilla, facial shape, evidence of teeth grinding and mouth breathing and tissue trauma like tongue scalloping. The dentist is in the front line for identifying all of these. For some children, expansion or correction of a malocclusion is recommended to help improve the airway, and this would involve wearing an appliance to help create more space in the mouth by widening the jaw.

Dental hygienists are also in the front line for screening of oral and airway health. Dental hygienists form a part of the oral health team in dentistry and orthodontics, supporting all aspects of oral and periodontal health. Some are also trained and skilled in myofunctional practice and principles, and may play a key role in screening for airway and sleep issues and subsequent myofunctional treatments.

Where airway issues are flagged for your child, airway-centric dental treatments in conjunction with the help of a myofunctional practitioner are a great combination, as they work on both structure and function. Your team, then, would be your dentist and your myofunctional practitioner. In other instances, your team may be an ENT with a dentist; in others an osteopath may become involved.

ORTHODONTIST

Orthodontics is a dental specialty that aims to prevent, diagnose and treat facial and dental irregularities such as malocclusion. However, its focus is not solely on teeth straightening, but is aligned with a philosophy for good airway development.[210]

Most of us are born with a less-than-ideal craniofacial skeleton, and we need assistance to get closer to what nature intended to open up the

210 Ibid.

airway.[211] Expansion is used to widen the palate or bring it forward, and this can mitigate airway problems (as it did for Jillian). While this is not a cure-all and may not be for everyone, it will be important for some.[212]

Although dentists and orthodontists recognise the importance of evaluating and treating OSA, some are yet to realise how well positioned they are for the prevention of sleep-disordered breathing. There is polarity in orthodontics, with some orthodontists advocating the role of orofacial muscles in the development, stability and maintenance of a healthy bite, while others do not. Some within the field are advocating for orthodontists to be on the front line with sleep disorders.[213] The approach makes a lot of sense.

Research is needed to work out how orthodontics may contribute to maximising facial growth from an early age so there is room for all of the teeth to come in without crowding. While orthodontists rarely see children before they start school, and many do not treat before highschool, for those who are embracing airway health and the importance of early jaw growth this practice may evolve and change over time.

Given this, it's best to be proactive and not wait until high school to see if your child has an airway issue that could be helped by orthodontic treatment. Try to find an orthodontist who will prioritise airway health and its development well before puberty. Your myofunctional practitioner or dentist may be able to help you find an airway-centric orthodontic practice.

Your orthodontist or dentist may refer you to a prosthodontist, 'the oral architect', who specialises in the restoration and replacement of teeth to improve or maintain oral function, health and appearance. A prosthodontist may play a key role for children whose airway is compromised

211 Sheldon et al., *Principles and Practice of Pediatric Sleep Medicine*.
212 Macario Camacho, Edward T. Chang, Sungjin A. Song, Jose Abdullatif, Soroush Zaghi, Paola Pirelli, Victor Certal and Christian Guilleminault, 'Rapid Maxillary Expansion for Pediatric Obstructive Sleep Apnea: A Systematic Review and Meta-Analysis', *The Laryngoscope* 127, no. 7 (2016), https://doi.org/10.1002/lary.26352.
213 Ruoff and Guilleminault, 'Orthodontics and Sleep-Disordered Breathing'.

by things like tooth agenesis (missing teeth) or tooth loss from trauma. Maintaining tooth integrity helps to maintain bone and jaw structure, and aiming for a full set of thirty-two teeth is a good target. For nine-year-old Emma, who has Koolen-de Vries syndrome, dental imaging revealed that she has seven teeth missing. This has significant implications for jaw growth and development, and Emma will need help from a prosthodontist to assist her jaw development and oral function.

The prosthodontist's role as the oral architect of the dental team means that they develop treatment plans and synchronise treatment sequences with dental and medical specialists in order to provide the most comprehensive care to patients.

EAR, NOSE AND THROAT SPECIALIST (ENT)

ENTs provide precision diagnosis to identify the root causes of SDB. They can view the whole of your child's upper airway, from the front of the face to the larynx, to look for potential obstructions and disruptions in the upper airway. This can be done while your child is awake or asleep.

An airway-focused ENT will consider:

- Jaw size and shape
- Signs of swelling, inflammation or obstruction in the airway (such as enlarged tonsils or narrow airway)
- Signs of teeth grinding
- Tissue restrictions that may affect the way the muscles function (such as tongue-tie)
- Otitis media or middle ear effusion
- Reflux or other gastrointestinal disturbances
- Allergies

Once an issue is identified, the ENT can recommend and provide treatment, which may be medication based or surgical. Simple nasal irrigation practices like 'Flo' or use of 'Breathe Right' strips (a nasal dilation system) may be recommended. These can significantly improve breathing, and very quickly. The 'Flo' system has a paediatric nozzle fitting. An ENT can also recommend medications for allergy or to reduce irritated tissues in the airway.

An ENT may refer you on to a dentist, orthodontist, audiologist, myofunctional practitioner or speech pathologist, depending on their findings.

Three-year-old Ryan was socially shy and his communication was about twelve months behind where it should be. He wasn't sleeping well, waking regularly in the middle of the night and struggling to get back to sleep. Ryan was a habitual mouth breather and his nose was always blocked.

When Ryan saw an ear, nose and throat specialist, the ENT was concerned about the cat sleeping on Ryan's bed every night. The ENT advised washing the bedclothes and soft toys in very hot water to remove allergens or particles like dust or pet dander and for Ryan to shower before bed to minimise any allergen exposure from the day. This all contributed to clearing Ryan's airway. Within four weeks, by fixing the issue that was leading to poor airway health and a poor breathing pattern, Ryan was as good as gold! In this instance he was referred for allergy testing and it turned out that the cat was not responsible for Ryan's issues; the culprit was an environmental allergen, pollen. Quite apart from the potential to cause an allergic reaction, however, pet movements and noises can disrupt sleep, so it's best to avoid pets sleeping on your child's bed.

If your ENT believes tonsils and adenoids are blocking or narrowing your child's airway and disrupting sleep, surgery may be recommended. For middle ears that are constantly filled with fluid, the ENT may insert grommets into the eardrums to provide drainage of the middle ear fluid. However, these problems also benefit from myo intervention in order to mobilise the muscles in the back of the throat where the drainage tubes from the ears are situated and where drainage naturally occurs. So, your team, then, would be your ENT, myofunctional practitioner and audiologist for regular monitoring of hearing and middle ear fluid.

ALLERGIST/IMMUNOLOGIST

When trying to find out exact causes of a blocked nose or airway issue, allergists and immunologists perform tests. They will be able to identify any allergy that may underpin airway problems. If they find an allergy, they can then offer ways to decrease symptoms that help kids breathe better.

The skin prick test is the most common way to identify potential allergies. The allergen test introduces small amounts of suspected allergens onto, and just below, the surface of the skin, with the number of pricks performed depending on how many allergens are being tested. Once the results of the test have been recorded, the nurse may apply a steroid ointment to help soothe any itchiness. Any allergies identified may then be treated by recommendation of the allergist, which could be via nasal spray, dust elimination in the home environment or a course of desensitisation. As we saw in Ryan's case, removal of allergens reduces irritants to the nasal passages and promotes ideal breathing throughout the day. This then supports an open airway and nasal breathing during sleep.

GASTROENTEROLOGIST

It is not uncommon for kids with airway obstruction to experience gastrointestinal issues.[214] The two are interrelated: research has shown that treating a patient's underlying sleep disorder may result in improvement in their gastrointestinal symptoms, while control of gastrointestinal disease states will result in improved sleep quality.

---

214 V. Khanijow, P. Prakash, H.A. Emsellem, M.L. Borum, D.B. Doman, 'Sleep Dysfunction and Gastrointestinal Diseases', *Gastroenterol Hepatol (N Y)* 11, no. 12 (2015):817–25.

If your child has a digestive system, liver or nutritional problem, a paediatric gastroenterologist has the expertise to diagnose and treat it. These problems in children are often quite different from those seen in adults, making specialised training and expertise in paediatric gastroenterology important. Paediatric gastroenterologists treat children from the newborn period through to the teen years. They will diagnose and treat issues like bleeding from the gastrointestinal tract, lactose intolerance, food allergies or intolerances, severe or complicated gastroesophageal reflux disease, inflammatory bowel disease, short bowel syndrome, liver disease, acute or chronic abdominal pain, vomiting, chronic constipation, chronic or severe diarrhoea, pancreatic insufficiency (including cystic fibrosis) and pancreatitis, nutritional problems (including malnutrition, failure to thrive, and obesity) and feeding disorders, all of which may have a reciprocal relationship with sleep disorders.

NEUROLOGIST/PAEDIATRIC NEUROLOGIST

A neurologist is a doctor who deals with diseases and conditions that affect the nervous system such as seizure disorders, febrile convulsions, epilepsy, medical aspects of head injuries, brain tumours, cerebral palsy, muscular dystrophy and neuromuscular disorders. If any of these are an issue for your child, your GP or paediatrician may ask a neurologist for an evaluation.

>> children with muscle weakness are at risk of airway collapsibility

This may be important for sleep, because children with muscle weakness are at risk of airway collapsibility.[215] Kids who experience pain from muscle contractures will also experience fragmented, interrupted sleep. A neurologist is therefore in a prime position to identify and treat kids at risk of sleep and airway problems related to neuromuscular conditions, brain disorders and diseases.

215 Guilleminault and Huang, 'From Oral Facial Dysfunction to Dysmorphism and the Onset of Pediatric OSA'.

SURGEON

A range of surgeons may be on your child's sleep team, whether an ENT specialist, paediatric dentist, paediatric surgeon, oral and maxillofacial surgeon, prosthodontist or a specialist team when dealing with craniofacial syndromes, anatomical and muscle tone anomalies or genetic disorders. Children with craniofacial disorders have multiple problems that require the expertise of a team who can support the child and family throughout all stages of development with the minimum physical, emotional and financial strain. For many surgical interventions are required.

'Craniofacial disorder' is a broad term that describes malformations of the face, which lead to problems with feeding, breathing, sleep and speech and language development. An example is cleft palate. Surgery can occur as early as three months and usually ends by twelve months, although secondary or further surgeries are sometimes needed down the track, along with regular developmental checks. The team is usually hospital based and often consists of a plastic surgeon, ENT, paediatric dentist, orthodontist, audiologist, geneticist, nurses, psychologist, social worker, speech pathologist, occupational therapist, physiotherapist, dietician and more.

Early treatment with an interdisciplinary team promotes and facilitates the best development for children with these conditions. Correcting physical abnormalities helps to minimise development of irregular compensatory behaviours and can maximise best conditions for growth in the upper airway. For instance, a narrow upper jaw can be widened or a tongue tie released to support optimum conditions for development.

PSYCHIATRIST

There is a strong relationship between mental health issues and sleep disorders. A psychiatrist is a medical doctor who specialises in mental health. When your child requires a prescription for medication in addition to counselling to deal with emotional or behavioural issues, that's when a psychiatrist can help. Your psychiatrist may also help with a differential diagnosis, meaning that they can look at a full range of symptoms and decide what diagnosis is consistent with your child's difficulties.

Depending on your child's needs, there may be a case for taking medication, but this should only ever follow expert medical advice. Over-the-counter medications, while tempting for a short-term solution, can exacerbate sleep problems. No over-the-counter medicines are appropriate as they can induce other issues. For example, giving your child sleep medication may cause them to wake (after falling asleep) and not get back to sleep. It may even have the opposite effect and stop them falling asleep.

>> Myofunctional practitioners perform a detailed assessment and diagnosis of the functions of the mouth, face, throat and oral habits

MYOFUNCTIONAL PRACTITIONER

Myofunctional practitioners perform a detailed assessment and diagnosis of the functions of the mouth, face, throat and oral habits. Once the assessment and diagnosis is completed, a myofunctional practitioner will design a program to correct oral rest postures, improve the strength, tone and range of movement of the muscles of the face, mouth and throat, correct head and neck posture, address all orofacial functions and eliminate harmful habits like thumb or finger-sucking. These functions are examined in relation to your child's upper airway health and any impact on sleep quality.

Your myofunctional practitioner will design the best possible therapy approach relevant to the age and interests of your child and based on the severity and nature of their symptoms. Each individual is different and therapy will be designed to integrate with any existing medical, dental, physical or behavioural conditions. Where sleep quality is affected, myofunctional therapy is therefore an important adjunctive treatment for sleep disorders like OSA and SBD.[216]

216 Leila Keirandish-Gozal, 'Morbidity Related Biomarkers in Pediatric Obstructive Sleep Apnea', *World Sleep Society Conference* (Prague, 2017).

If your child is diagnosed with an orofacial myofunctional disorder, this is when myo-correct comes in. The aim of myo-correct is to develop awareness and control of the muscles of the mouth, face and throat. Myo-correct is an intensive approach with an initial focus on exercises that act as a stepping stone to functions already mentioned earlier in this chapter. The goal is to train the muscles to develop new rest and movement habits during breathing, swallowing and chewing, that become automatic. This new way of using the muscles will then replace the old way. It is critical, however, that the end point of therapy is function and for this to happen there must be specificity in myo which focusses away from exercises and onto function. [217,218] Exercises are often easy; the challenge is developing new daily habits.

Myo-correct starts with correction of mouth breathing and oral habits like thumb or dummy sucking, as, until these are corrected, they will interfere with successful retraining of atypical muscles patterns. Getting nose breathing right may require medical help, while children with very narrow jaw structures may need the intervention of a dentist or orthodontist to widen the upper jaw. Once the oral habits and nose breathing are corrected, a series of foundation movements of the face, mouth and throat are provided to increase awareness and control of the muscles.

If there is any other structural issue that is getting in the way of retraining muscles, then it may also need medical intervention (such as treating allergies, removal of tonsils or adenoids or correcting a tongue-tie). Your myofunctional practitioner will guide you to the best practitioners for these issues. However, even where medical intervention is required for your child, like grommets, adenotonsillectomy or frenectomy (tongue-tie release), there will still be a period of muscle retraining required to improve mouth, face and throat muscle function, both before or after surgery.

---

217 Heather M. Clark, 'Neuromuscular Treatments for Speech and Swallowing', *American Journal of Speech-Language Pathology* 12, no. 4 (2003), https://doi.org/10.1044/1058-0360(2003/086).

218 Heather Clark, 'Motor Learning and Neuromuscular Principles: Applications to Myofunctional Disorder', in *The 1st AAMS Congress*, (Los Angeles, 2015).

Myo-correct can even help to rule a problem in or out. I have seen many cases in the clinic where a tongue looks and behaves in a very restricted way due to a tongue-tie, but after a myo-correct program the tongue is able to achieve normal function. For this reason, it's important not to jump to conclusions around the need for surgical intervention. Sometimes a long period of evaluation is required before suggesting a surgical solution.

>> 'Chip away, a little everyday'. That's how kids in my clinic learn their myo mantra and get really good at it

The goal of both myo-optimise and myo-correct is to develop great breathing, chewing, swallowing and oral rest postures, which support and promote craniofacial growth, maintain and stabilise occlusion, promote great dental health and optimise the development and function of the airway. These new skills do not develop overnight. While exercises can be learnt very quickly, learning to chew, swallow and breathe in a new way often takes six to twelve months of consistent chipping away, just like learning a musical instrument. As we say in my clinic: 'Chip away, a little everyday'. That's how kids in my clinic learn their myo mantra and get really good at it.

A myofunctional practitioner could be a speech pathologist, dental hygienist, physiotherapist or occupational therapist who has done additional study and training in myofunctional practice. Dentists, orthodontists and other health practitioners also do the training so that they enhance their understanding of myo, but very few do the actual therapy. The background of your myofunctional practitioner will determine the scope of the myo-correct program and whether your child also goes on to work with voice, resonance and speech – skills which are within the scope of practice for a speech pathologist, for example, but not a physiotherapist or dental hygienist.

You will find a wide range of skills among myofunctional practitioners, and there is active progression towards creating a universal standard for myofunctional competencies and clinical practice.

BREATHING EDUCATOR

Once a dysfunctional breathing habit has set in, correction often requires expert help. This involves developing new, healthy breathing patterns during sleep, everyday activities and exercise.

>> Myo and breathing re-education go hand in hand for management of airway problems and airway-related sleep disorders

A skilled breathing educator will be able to help with this. Buteyko breathing is a well-known breathing re-education system that can help to correct aberrant breathing habits like mouth breathing and other forms of dysfunctional breathing.[219] Some myofunctional practitioners are dual trained as breathing educators and can provide breathing correction concurrently to myo. Myo and breathing re-education go hand in hand for management of airway problems and airway-related sleep disorders. Many allied health practitioners have also added the Buteyko breathing skills to their toolbox and there are many trained breathing educators worldwide. For your child, and perhaps your whole family, it's best to choose someone who has good experience with a range of patients and who is happy to work with other team members to develop your child's upper airway health.

Correcting breathing patterns may not be as simple as retraining habits, so it is important to uncover whether or not there are underlying medical factors associated with dysfunctional breathing. For example, a child with a bead stuck in the nose, nasal polyps or a deviated septum will be unable to breathe well due to anatomical constraints, and no amount of breathing retraining will correct it. This will require intervention from an ENT specialist first rather than a breathing specialist.

219 'The Complete Buteyko Method For Children and Teenagers', Buteyko Clinic International, accessed January 1, 2018, http://buteykoclinic.com/buteykochildren.

SPEECH PATHOLOGIST

Speech pathologists diagnose and treat communication and swallowing disorders. While their scope of practice is very broad, those who work with medical and dental specialists focus more on the upper airway functions.

A speech pathologist might become involved with a baby's airway development or function in a NICU or other hospital setting, where they diagnose and treat feeding and swallowing disorders for medically compromised babies and children. For some children, treatment using oro-motor therapy approaches is used to assist development of the mouth and face and improve feeding and swallowing so that safe eating and drinking is possible. The primary focus in these settings is safe nutritional intake.

It is also a prime opportunity to begin myo at a pace and difficulty level that a child can cope with easily. Some speech pathologists are also trained as myofunctional practitioners, which enables them to work closely with medical and dental specialists in a team working towards optimum upper airway health and development. Interestingly, when working with swallowing, the speech pathologist's role is to help a patient swallow safely and is all about closing the airway, whereas when working to improve breathing during sleep, the role is to open the airway.[220] Both of course are critical to health.

In Brazil, speech-language pathologists (SLPs) who are trained in orofacial myofunctional therapy play a very important role in the management of patients with airway related sleep disorders, providing therapy to 'keep the airway open'. It is a non-invasive and educational treatment. Brazilian SLPs have an official certification to allow them to do this work, and are laying down the footprints for other speech pathologists worldwide to follow.

---

220 E. Bianchini, 'Pathways to Update Standards of Care: How Myofunctional Therapy Works in OSA', AAMS workshop, pre *World Sleep Society Conference* (Prague, 2017).

>> **Because speech pathologists are involved from birth onwards, they are at the front line for identifying signs of sleep disorders in children, in particular those related to airway**

Because speech pathologists are involved with tiny little humans from birth and onwards, they are at the front line for identifying and flagging signs and symptoms of sleep disorders, in children, particular those related to airway.[221] Again, the importance of airway has not filtered through to all speech pathologists worldwide, but the seeds are being sown.

OCCUPATIONAL THERAPIST

Occupational therapists (OTs) help children achieve their developmental milestones such as fine motor skills and hand-eye coordination. They also educate and involve parents and carers to facilitate normal development and learning for kids.

Children with compromised early development and disabilities will benefit from the input of an occupational therapist as part of their overall care. Again, because OTs are involved with tiny little humans from birth, they are at the front line for identifying and flagging signs and symptoms of sleep problems, in particular those related to airway.

PHYSIOTHERAPIST

Paediatric physiotherapy provides assessment, diagnosis and therapy for a child's movement and posture, aiming for best muscle and joint function in a growing child's body, including head and neck posture which is critical for health and function of the upper airway. Physio may be required to help kids move and maintain alignment as well as reminders and good postural habit development.

Unlike adults, who have completed their growth period, children may have specific needs relating to their ongoing physical development that can benefit from a paediatric physiotherapist. In the growing child, bone

221 Moore, 'Sleep Disorders are in Your Face'.

growth may outperform muscle growth, and problems can arise that require an understanding of all such factors. A paediatric physiotherapist's skill with posture, fascia release and breathing may be particularly helpful for children whose airway issues are interfering with sleep.

DIETICIAN

A paediatric dietician specialises in creating and evaluating nutrition programs and policies for children from infancy to eighteen years of age. Some of the areas they can help with include special nutrition care for premature babies, food intolerances, low-grade chronic stress and advice on foods that may lead to sleep onset problems (such as sweets, sugary drinks or foods that contain artificial flavours or colourings). Some children may have sensitivities to certain foods, such as dairy or wheat, which can stimulate their brain or upset their digestive system e.g. cause reflux, which may interfere staying asleep. Some may be low on iron or other essential vitamins, or perhaps they have fallen into the overweight zone and it is impacting their airway. A dietician's expertise may be invaluable for these kids.

CHIROPRACTOR

Chiropractic care may be helpful to address musculoskeletal issues that interfere with a comfortable night's sleep, by treating tension sites with gentle care. Many families opt for regular chiropractic care. The most important thing to understand is whether the treatment is helping to address the underlying cause or provide symptom relief. This determines who else needs to be on your sleep team.

A chiropractic treatment may include soft tissue massage, mobilisations or gentle adjustments to relieve stress on a child's spine and increase flexibility and movement in the joints. This is important in the rib and chest area for breathing, as decreased flexibility in this area restricts the inflation capability of the chest wall. While this might not be noticeable when your child is awake, the increased energy required to take a full deep breath takes its toll during sleep, creating restlessness.

>> When sleep problems are resolvable by adapting your child's behaviour, environment and routine, it can be relatively easy for parents to solve on their own

Who can help with disordered sleep?

When sleep problems are resolvable by adapting your child's behaviour, environment and routine, it can be relatively easy for parents to solve on their own without professional expertise. These issues come under the banner of disordered sleep. However, stubborn behavioural issues may require support. If you can't crack the nut on your own, persist and find a health professional who can help and support you with helpful behavioural strategies. These may take time to establish, and some children may be harder nuts to crack than others.[222] Tricky environmental spaces may also require the creative brain of a third party. So, when sleep problems exist because of sleep hygiene issues, routines, habits, behaviour or environment, the following professionals might be able to help.

SLEEP SPECIALIST

If a sleep specialist has completed sleep investigations for your child and ruled out sleep disorders, they will give you advice or guidance about possible adaptions to behaviour, habits, routines and environment. This may come in the form of counselling or a referral to another specialist like a paediatrician, psychologist or psychiatrist.

NEUROPSYCHOLOGIST/PSYCHOLOGIST/BEHAVIOURAL PSYCHOLOGIST/PSYCHIATRIST

Because we live in a world where chronic low-grade stress is the norm, a psychologist or psychiatrist can be very helpful for teaching families and kids how to develop skills to 'defrag' from the push and pull of daily living. To defrag means to unravel the emotional tensions that arise from busy schedules and lives and unexpected challenges.

222 Sarah Blunden, 'Behavioural Sleep Disorders'.

Kids with special needs or disabilities, along with those living with chronic pain or with serious illnesses, may also benefit from the skills of a paediatric psychologist or psychiatrist. Difficulty regulating behaviour and emotions goes hand in hand with sleep disorders. Often, behaviour and fractiousness resolves when the sleep issue resolves (and vice versa). Psychological support can also be helpful for kids who have patterns of unhealthy or unhelpful emotional responses that have become habitual. The same goes for situations where there is family conflict or unrest. Children can benefit from outside support during these times as much as adults. Cognitive behaviour therapy is a widely accepted intervention that can help kids with anxiety or stress.

When kids' sleep is compromised, classroom problems can arise as problem solving, reasoning, focus and self-regulation are all challenged. A neuropsychologist or psychologist will be able to do a detailed assessment of a child's abilities. Learning focus and attention issues can resolve when the sleep problem is resolved. The classroom teacher is a key front-line person who may recognise a child's sleep problem before anyone else.

As mentioned above, a psychiatrist is a medical doctor who specialises in mental health and can prescribe medication if required.

SLEEP COACH

If all possible medical issues have been treated and your child's sleep behaviour is still resistant to change, a professional sleep coach may be able to help in your home. There are many sleep coaches out there, and it will be important to find one with a philosophy and approach that fits your family. For babies, I like Tracy Newberry's approach of teaching sleep with love, kindness and the utmost respect, and I've shared some of Tracy's wisdom in Appendix A.[223] If you are suffering from the exhaustion of relentless sleep deprivation and the anguish of

---

223 Tracy Newberry, 'Teaching Sleep With Love, Kindness And The Utmost Respect', http://www.happybabyandme.com/.

being a parent in this situation, you could search for someone in your area who has a similar approach to Tracy or someone that aligns with your philosophies on parenting.

THIRD-PARTY MAGIC

As mentioned in Chapter 4, you could have your own 'home grown' sleep coach, meaning a family member or friend who is happy to help break resistant sleep habits and help create new routines.

CHILDCARE PROFESSIONAL

Many childcare professionals have a special knack with kids and managing their shenanigans. So if you have a trusted helper like a babysitter or nanny, why not enlist their help to get on top of a disordered sleep issue or to help rearrange a sleeping environment? You could also ask your kid's childcare worker or preschool teacher for input, as they will be familiar with your child and their behaviours and may have some fresh insights into what could work best for them.[224]

INTERIOR DESIGNER

Don't be shy about asking for support to help you make the sleeping environment just right for your child. If you need help designing a room and creating a sleep sanctuary to set your little ones up for blissful sleep, ask an interior designer.

CHIROPRACTOR

Alongside helping with musculoskeletal issues, chiropractors can also recommend mattresses and pillows that are specially designed to support growing bodies and offer advice on correct sleeping position.

---

224 Claire Broad, *How to Be the Big Person Your Little Person Needs* (Sydney, N.S.W.: The OMNE Group, 2015).

Who can help with babies?

OBSTETRICIAN/GYNAECOLOGIST

These specialists provide medical and surgical care to women and have particular expertise in pregnancy, childbirth, and disorders of the reproductive system. They are in the prime position to identify a mother whose breathing is compromised during pregnancy and at risk of SDB or OSA, which may compromise the baby's development in utero and lead to possible premature birth.[225,226]

In a perfect world, kids at risk would be identified in utero. Educating mothers to be on the importance of upper airway health may provide an additional layer of health vigilance for mum and her developing baby. Foetal echography allows the assessment of the baby's movements in utero, including sucking and swallowing movements. Babies at risk could be identified before birth so that early myo can be flagged to commence as soon after birth as possible.

Premature babies born to mothers with compromised airways do not have a mature system for breathing, sucking and swallowing at birth. Obstetricians and gynaecologists may be in a position to flag these issues as early as possible.

NEONATOLOGIST

Neonatologists diagnose and treat newborns with conditions such as breathing disorders, infections and birth defects. They coordinate care and medically manage premature or critically ill newborns or those in need of surgery.

Neonatologists are in a prime position to screen at-risk kids from the earliest possible age and activate support plans to help mums breast-

225 Children's National Health System, 'Preterm Infants Have Narrowed Upper Airways, Which May Explain Higher Obstructive Sleep Apnea Risk', ScienceDaily, accessed January 7, 2018, https://www.sciencedaily.com/releases/2017/12/171223134801.htm.

226 Smitthimedhin, 'MRI Determination of Volumes for the Upper Airway and Pharyngeal Lymphoid Tissue in Preterm and Term Infants'.

feed, including possible frenectomy. Where breastfeeding is not possible, they may be in a position to encourage and coordinate support for early oral reflex stimulation, which will encourage the essential movements and strengthening of the face, mouth, tongue and jaw.

Abnormalities of sleep breathing can develop very early in life, and if risk factors are recognised in childhood and treated early, babies, particularly premature babies, can get a great start to airway health.

PAEDIATRIC GASTROENTEROLOGIST

Paediatric gastroenterologists treat children from the newborn period through to the teen years. They will diagnose and treat a range of issues as mentioned above on page 185.

LACTATION CONSULTANT

Remember how important it is to kick start a baby's muscle and facial development with breastfeeding? When things don't get off to a great start, International Board-Certified Lactation Consultants can assist mums to develop effective breastfeeding and identify problems that may be interfering, such as low muscle tone, poor feeding technique, difficulty with suck-swallow-breathe coordination, small mouth or a tongue-tie.

Some babies' feeding problems do not show up until three to twelve months after birth. For example, a mum's copious milk supply can mask some early feeding problems because the baby is getting enough to eat and gaining weight even though their technique is not optimal.

IBCLCs can also help babies with bottle-feeding and other alternatives required at this time. 'Body Workers' can also be invaluable to help with developing postural control and awareness.

OSTEOPATH

Osteopathy involves using soft manipulation techniques to reduce or remove tensions in the skull and body, correcting postural alignment difficulties that can arise during gestation and birth.

While it is physiologically normal for a baby to wake up at night, other elements can sometimes worsen waking and contribute to sleep disorder symptoms. Contributing problems can be things like poor head position, cranial tensions, torticollis, or digestive system disorders like reflux and colic, or tongue-tie.

Osteopathic examination can identify tensions in the body that may be disturbing sleeping patterns. For example, some children can have over-stimulated nervous systems, which mean they are unable to 'switch off' and go to sleep. While routine and environment are critical to help a child relax, unresolved muscle tension in the head, neck and body can perpetuate difficulty going to sleep. An osteopath may help by reducing this tension through different manual therapy techniques.

Many lactation-specialist GPs refer regularly to osteopaths for assistance with young babies establishing breastfeeding.[227]

CHILDCARE PROFESSIONAL

As with small children, many childcare professionals have a way with babies and managing their shenanigans, and may be able to help you with your baby's sleep routine and environment or provide support and advice in the case of disordered sleep. General advice around behaviour management can be invaluable.

---

227 Juliette Herzhaft-Le Roy, Marianne Xhignesse and Isabelle Gaboury, 'Efficacy of an Osteopathic Treatment Coupled With Lactation Consultations for Infants' Biomechanical Sucking Difficulties', *Journal of Human Lactation* 33, no. 1 (2016), https://doi.org/10.1177/0890334416679620.

SLEEP COACH

Particularly with babies, it can be very helpful to employ a professional sleep coach when starting new sleep habits, routines and behaviours. See more in Appendix A (see page 215).

ALLIED HEALTH PRACTITIONERS

All allied health practitioners may have a role with babies as previously outlined, including:

- Speech pathologist
- Dietician
- Occupational therapist
- Physiotherapist

These allied health practitioners may work in medical settings where they care regularly for babies, particularly medically compromised babies. In a perfect world, all medical, allied medical and childcare professionals would work as a team to identify all and any kids at risk of sleep disorders or disordered sleep and provide the required treatment. Ideally, they would have done additional study in myo to best assist a baby's airway development.

How to choose the right specialist for your child

Remember Jillian from the beginning of this chapter? When we were investigating her sleep and airway issues, an acquaintance of Jillian's family, who happened to be a paediatric dentist, disagreed with the suggested approach to improving Jillian's airway, even though it was the parents' decision and choice after being offered several options to improve Jillian's airway. Not only that, she felt so strongly about it that, even though Jillian was not a patient of hers, she wrote a letter stating her disapproval.

Because sleep medicine is an emerging discipline, there remains some polarised thinking among the medical and dental communities when it comes to diagnosis and treatment of airway related disorders. This is one reason why it can be difficult to choose and find experts to work with your kids.

Thankfully, the number of medical specialists who recognise the importance of sleep and airway health is growing. This trend was apparent at the recent World Sleep Society congress in Prague, 2017, where more than forty leaders in the field of sleep medicine acknowledged the role of myofunctional therapy in the management of airway-related sleep disorders. The field of sleep medicine is active in research, and this research is much needed to facilitate our knowledge and clinical practice guidelines across all medical and dental disciplines involved in caring for kids with sleep problems and to ensure that kids are getting the treatment they need as early as possible.

Finding the right specialist or specialist team for your family can be as simple as checking to see if your doctor, dentist, specialist or allied health practitioner has sleep health on their radar, and if their thinking and treatment approach aligns with your child's sleep and airway needs.

When finding a medical and allied health support team for your child, chances are that you already have concerns and have identified red flags for sleep and airway problems. You will need to explain what your concerns are and why you want advice.

The following questions should help you discern whether your practitioner is 'sleep and airway interested'. You can ask these kinds of questions when you call to make enquiries or during a routine visit to your health practitioner. If you are asking your GP or paediatrician for a referral to a specialist or allied health practitioner, you could first ask them these questions in order to get the right recommendation. I suggest that you don't ask all of these questions – just choose one or two depending on who you are seeing and the reason for your visit.

Before asking your questions, you can share your concerns by saying, "I'm concerned about my child because he/she: is not getting enough sleep *or* not getting the right kind of sleep *or* not waking refreshed *or* their behaviour makes it seem like they are tired."

- Does your clinic use a sleep screening questionnaire?
- Does your clinic consider both quantity and quality of sleep?
- Are sleep issues screened when a child has ADHD-like symptoms?
- Does your clinic work with and refer to other professionals who may assist with a sleep or airway diagnosis?
- Is polysomnography available if necessary? Or is accurate home testing available?
- If you are seeing a dentist or orthodontist: Does your evaluation include, teeth, jaws and airway health?
- Does your treatment philosophy provide early treatment for symptoms of sleep or airway problems, or a 'wait, watch and see' approach?
- Who else is on your 'sleep and airway' team if there is a sleep problem? ENT? Dentist? Allergist? Psychologist? Myofunctional practitioner?
- If not your clinic, who can you recommend for help with sleep and airway issues?

Once you have had a chance to meet and you feel comfortable that your dental, medical or allied health practitioners will consider your concerns about the red flags you have found, you have discovered the 'right fit' for your family.

Working in partnership with your specialist team

If you work with a medical and allied health team, they will help you address your child's sleep disorder or disordered sleep.

However, regardless of how good your specialist team is, you will always be the most important member of your child's team – the chief lifeguard. By being aware and proactive you will identify issues early and ensure they do not have the chance to develop into long-term disorders. A specialist can advise you on what action to take and how to take that action, but much of it is up to you to manage and follow through at home.

Consider Harry-the-Champion. Harry was six years old when his mum came to me. She had made some acute and important observations and thought Harry's myofunctional issues might be connected to Harry's disrupted sleep and account for some daytime behavioural and personality traits. She was a clever, observant mother, and it turned out she was right. Harry's muscles were weak and not in good shape; he was a mouth breather and had been a snorer since the age of two. His upper jaw was very narrow.

Harry went on to participate in eight weeks of 'myo-correct' therapy. While much of it was very challenging in the beginning because his muscles did not want to cooperate, Harry very quickly became the poster boy for myofunctional therapy. Harry's whole family did myo at home. His mum was so good at engaging the whole family that the new chewing, swallowing and breathing patterns became the norm for them all. The exercise challenges became a point of pride for young Harry, who beat the existing clinic record for the 'water trap' exercise by holding it for eighteen minutes, a record previously held at sixteen minutes by a ten-year-old boy! Yes, that's a long time to hold a sip of water to the roof of your mouth. He beat other records, too. Harry really was a champion.

In just eight sessions of in-clinic therapy and great home practice, eighty-five per cent of Harry's night-time and daytime symptoms disappeared. He became more self-assured and was very proud of his achievements. However, we were not quite finished. Regular myo follow-up is required over time to ensure the new habits stabilise into the new norm. In addition, medical and dental follow-ups were also required to manage due to a possible tongue movement restriction, allergy and a narrow-vaulted palate.

While there are many kids who have similar issues to Harry, not everyone has such a good track record with home practice. Family life can be chaotic and fitting in myo can be a challenge. Consequently, their progress is slower. However, Harry showed us what is possible when the whole family is on board. By all accounts they had a lot of fun. Most kids and families take up to twelve months to fully integrate new habits and skills into daily life.

> **>> You can have a profound effect on your child's life by helping them achieve essential, deep sleep and optimal airway health**

Of course, much about a child's airway health can also be influenced by other factors like nutrition, exercise, stress, and exposure to pollutants. Remember epigenetics – the lifestyle factors under our control that can influence gene expression? By managing all these factors well and prioritising sleep, you can change the course of your child's future. We may all be stuck with inherited genes, but we can still influence the course of the development of our facial morphology and airway. Knowing what you *can* influence, including which experts can help you, puts you in a great position as your child's lifeguard. You can have a profound effect on your child's life by helping them achieve essential, deep sleep and optimal airway health.

There is always more than one lifeguard at the beach. Others may take turns to be 'on watch' and contribute in different ways to your child's care. Because every child's (and every family's) needs are different, there are times when a bigger team may be required, particularly for kids with diagnosed syndromes or disabilities. The medical team will be working with you to get your child's sleep formula just right. But as the parent, your lifeguard role is continuous. Your kids will see the best improvement if you are consistent and thorough with following up on advice from your expert team. In playing this lifeguard role to get your child's sleep and airway functioning just right, you can have a profound effect on their developing nervous system and every aspect of health, growth and development. You can set them up for life of health and happiness and the full expression of their IQ – and help them grow into the very best version of themselves.

Conclusion: What's next?

'We can make a better world by empowering children's sleep.'

– DR ROSALIE SILVESTRI[228]

Together we've been on quite a journey, uncovering the true costs of sleep problems in sleep-wrecked kids and learning how to be lifeguards when it comes to their sleep and airway health. As you implement the advice shared in this book and work with your team of specialists, your child's sleep – and life – will continue to improve. Sleep matters a lot and so do parents.

So, what happens next?

We know that, as parents, our work is never truly over. Life is constantly changing, children are continually developing and we're unlikely to be able to sit down, put our feet up and tick 'fix my child's sleep' off the to-do list in a definitive way. So, I have three final pieces of wisdom for you as you move out of the sleep-wrecked phase: take your own sleep seriously, stay vigilant and spread the word.

Take your own sleep seriously

Parenting is, without a doubt, one of the most challenging roles in life. Even when children are pretty near perfect, they have good and bad days (just like parents do). On the bad days, it can sometimes be too much to bear. This is why, if you are going to be your child's lifeguard, you need your sleep just as much as your child needs theirs.

Many adults don't prioritise their own sleep. In Australia, the National Sleep Foundation's 2016 survey discovered that up to forty-five per cent

228 Rosalie Sivestri 'Introduction', in *World Sleep Society Conference* (Prague, 2017).

of Australian adults get an inadequate quality or quantity of sleep every night – and suffer the daytime consequences.[229]

It's not just kids who engage in night-time shenanigans. Adults tend to have a bit of a 'tough it out' approach to sleep. With burgeoning workloads, a desire to cram everything into one day, twenty-four-hour media and permanent access to the internet, people are sleeping less and less, with well over thirty per cent of adults in Western societies getting less sleep than they need.[230]

>> When you are sleep deprived, you will find it difficult to play the essential lifeguard role in your child's life

When you are sleep deprived, not only will you suffer from all the symptoms discussed in Chapter 1 – fatigue, inability to focus, erratic moods, physical aches and pains and more – you will find it difficult to play your essential lifeguard role in your child's life. You will have low energy or willpower to stick to the bedtime routine, deal with night-time shenanigans or even properly observe your kid's progress.

Remember Layla and Ben from Chapter 3? When their mum was completing the intake questionnaire, we also discovered that both parents were having sleepless nights. This increased parental tensions around everything from what to feed the kids to how to discipline them. On top of that, both parents were in full-time, high-powered jobs that required them to travel, so they had the added challenge of maintaining a routine for their children when one or both parents were absent. Anxiety and stress were frequent guests in their home, which further contributed to poor sleep and short tempers for everyone.

229 Robert Adams, Sarah Appleton, Anne Taylor, Doug McEvoy and Nick Antic, 'Report to the Sleep Health Foundation: 2016 Sleep Health Survey of Australian Adults', University of Adelaide, Adelaide Institute for Sleep Health (Adelaide, 2016), https://www.sleephealthfoundation.org.au/pdfs/surveys/SleepHealthFoundation–Survey.pdf.
230 Schoenborn and Adams, 'Health Behaviours Of Adults'.

These parents had to start prioritising their own sleep as well as their child's – and it's important that you do the same. If your sleep *quantity* is off, start going to bed a bit earlier to get those hours up. If your sleep *quality* is off, look at your own sleeping environment, bedtime routine and physical health. If you have a diagnosed sleep disorder, seek medical help as a top priority. If you're not much of a morning person, look at ways to nurture yourself so you are waking happy and calm and ready for the day. Minimising your own crankiness will have a flow-on effect for everyone around you, including your kids.

>> By becoming a good model of sleep literacy and sleep hygiene, you can help your child sleep better, too

Not only will better sleep mean you can be the parent, partner and lifeguard you need to be, a secondary benefit is that you will act as a model for your child. Kids are constantly learning from those around them, and you are one of their biggest influences. They learn by watching what you do rather than listening to what you say. By becoming a good model of sleep literacy and sleep hygiene, you can help your child sleep better, too.

Stay vigilant

If things have improved, parents can quickly forget the pain, frustration and despair caused by sleep problems. It's just like 'pain amnesia' following childbirth, where a mother is so in love and so completely immersed with the new baby that she forgets the pain very quickly.

Once you are getting your sleep again, you will very quickly forget the trauma of existing in a sleep fog or the frayed nerves from living with a tired-wired child. You will quickly return to enjoying your child, watching them grow well and learn to their full IQ potential. And so you should!

But as you know, your job is not really finished. You will always be the lifeguard of sleep (and many other things) for your child. Therefore, it's helpful to check in every so often to ensure that everything is still going smoothly for their sleep.

This doesn't need to be extreme, but it's important to regularly monitor your child's old symptoms and not to let good habits slip. You can have a checklist on the fridge or maintain your bedtime routine charts and stickers to keep everything on your radar.

From time to time, it will also be valuable to revisit the assessments from Chapter 3 in order to measure improvements or catch any new red flags. Is your child still exhibiting any sleep red flags? Are they getting the right number of hours of sleep per day? Do they go to sleep quickly and rest quietly? Do they sleep through the night? Do they wake up refreshed and stay alert and happy for the day? How about their behaviour, environment or routine? Are they experiencing any medical and dental issues? Is their growth and development on track? Have there been life events and challenges that have created a setback? Or caused relapse into old habits?

Revisiting these questions on a semi-regular basis can help everyone stay on track.

Spread the word

With all of the information you have at your fingertips, taking charge of your child's health and life trajectory will become a responsibility you can enjoy. You have the tools you need to create the right opportunity for your child to develop to their very best version of themselves. Our kids are the leaders of the future, and building that future starts at home. Truly, every child deserves to get the sleep they need, every night.

So, why not share your new-found knowledge with other parents and help them build a bright future for their kids, too? Keep your lifeguard cap on for all the kids around you, and talk to other parents and friends who might be struggling with their own kids' sleep. Take every opportunity to let people

>> parents tell me on a daily basis, 'Why didn't someone tell me this before?'

know about your story, how you discovered a way to rescue your family from the clutches of poor sleep and what a big difference it has made to family happiness, because there are millions out there who are suffering unnecessarily.

I hear parents telling me on a daily basis, 'Why didn't someone tell me this before?' From my own experience as a mother, if I'd had help when my kids were little it would have saved us from some heartache and significant loss of sleep. Personally, I can't think of anything better to do with my career right now than help parents make a difference in their families' daily lives and their kids' future health and wellbeing by solving sleep problems in a world where they pose major health and education issues that are not yet solved.

And who is better to spread the word than someone who has been there? Rather than give advice, talk about what you did to fix your child's sleep and the results you've seen. Your personal story is powerful and, while other parents may resist taking advice, if they hear your wonderful story it may inspire them to do the same for their family. Let's open the world's eyes to the truth about sleep!

>> you can be the tipping point – that "magic moment" when new ideas about sleep will spread like wildfire

I believe the parent network is phenomenal. There's a force of mums and dads the world around who want the best for their children and will do anything to make that happen. All they need is the right information. Perhaps you can be the tipping point[231] – that 'magic moment when new ideas about sleep will spread like wildfire'. When parents start working collaboratively, they are a force to be reckoned with.

231 Malcolm Gladwell, *The Tipping Point: How Little Things Can Make a Big Difference* (London: Abacus, 2000).

It just starts with a good night's sleep.

> Learn more about children and development in this fantastic TED Talk, which discusses a parent's role in helping children do well at school and life:
>
> https://www.ted.com/talks/helen_pearson_lessons_from_the_longest_study_on_human_development

Appendices

Appendix A: Building good sleep habits for babies

*'When babies don't sleep, seventy per cent of mothers have
aggressive thoughts and fantasies.'*

– DR O. BRUNI[232]

Sleep is essential to babies' brain development, helping babies learn to develop memories, rejuvenate from the day before and prepare for the day to come. Growth hormone (somatomedin) is released while babies are in deep sleep, ensuring they grow well. A well-slept baby is a happy baby.

However, overnight waking is a reality with babies, at least for a while. Newborns and young infants require a lot of attention through the night, as they need frequent feeding and nappy changes. 'The books' say that once your child is six to twelve months old they should be able to sleep through the night on their own, but many babies don't sleep through the night for the first twelve months. It's not uncommon for babies to have night-time feeds for their first year, with some continuing up to eighteen months.

When a baby is not sleeping well, it affects not just the baby but also family dynamics and parents' mental health. New mums are often exhausted and have limited support systems. Some even feel guilty if their child doesn't fit with the textbook or expected norms. It's hard to function at our best and be the parents we want to be when we are not getting the sleep we need, but with babies this can be a real Catch-22. How do you get the sleep you need when your baby is not sleeping?

232 Bruni, 'Insomnia: Clinical and Diagnostic Aspects'.

How to help your bub get a good night's sleep

Good sleep for a baby follows the same formula as everyone else's: quality plus quantity.

In a twenty-four-hour period, the ideal quantity is as follows:

AGE	SLEEP REQUIRED	
Newborn–2 months	16–18 hours	8–9 hours at night
		7–9 hours in naps throughout the day
2–4 months	14–16 hours	9–10 hours at night
		4–5 hours across 3 naps
4–6 months	14–15 hours	10 hours at night
		4–5 hours across 2–3 naps

How can you help with this? Setting up your baby's sleep environment and their routine, along with gentle nurturing, will help a lot.

Your baby's sleep environment

Sleep is not black or white, and babies wake for so many different reasons. When looking at baby's sleep, not only is it important to note what's typical for their age and how to set up and establish positive sleep habits and associations but also to consider and be respectful of their sleep environment.

Tracy Newberry is a sleep coach with a passion for helping babies learn to sleep well in a kind, loving way without using any crying. She has taught hundreds of parents how to help their littlies sleep well gently.

If you think babies are unaware of their environment and should be able to sleep anywhere, think again! Once Tracy helped a mum with her little boy who wasn't sleeping very well. On walking into the baby's room, the reason for his troubles was plain to Tracy. The family lived in a large house with the baby's room on the top floor. It was a massive room with a huge floor-to-ceiling window spanning an entire wall. Before the baby was born, this room was used as a storage room. However, this baby arrived early, and his parents didn't have the time to get it in order. They had even less time to work on it after his arrival, so the room was still a storage room. There were pots of paint on the floor, spare tiles piled high, tools and building equipment shoved in corners and a tall ladder leaning against a wall. While he was still too young to crawl and get into trouble with all the dangerous objects around him, the atmosphere in his room was not conducive to sleep at all.

Tracy moved this poor bub's nursery to a better room in the house, setting it up to be conducive to sleep with Feng Shui principles and introducing white noise and blackout blinds. She added a nap time and bedtime routine, making both easier. Tracy and his mum also looked at his awake times to find the ideal time he needed to be put down for a nap before becoming overtired, which was then making it harder to sleep. Mum invested in a high-quality mattress and bedding, corrected the temperature in the room, she chose the appropriate tog sleeping bag to use and dressed him in 100 per cent organic cotton for sleep times. Mum also doubled up on the nappies as often he would leak through (which then woke him up).

After this, he slept like a baby!

The environment in which your baby sleeps plays a significant part in how well they sleep. Often this is overlooked, but when we think about it logically, everything that affects an adults sleep affects a baby's sleep in just the same way.

You want your baby's room to feel peaceful, comforting and safe – a place to unwind. Here are some tips to achieve this:

Light

Light stimulates a baby's eyes to tell them it's time to wake up. Use blackout blinds on the windows and roll up a towel or blanket and place it outside at the foot of your baby's door to block out any light streaming in.

Make sure no visible lights are coming from your electrical appliances, such as your baby monitor, and cover any lights that could disturb your little one's sleep.

Noise

Just like us, surrounding noise can disturb a little one's sleep. Use white noise to mask your everyday household sounds as well as outdoor noise (dogs barking, sirens wailing), which could disrupt your little one's sleep.

White noise is repetitive and calming, often mimicking sounds of the womb, which can be incredibly soothing and help babies stay asleep for longer. An example of White Noise is sounds of a womb, heartbeat, fan, vacuum cleaner, rain, ocean, seashore, shushing or hushing and noise of a hairdryer.

White noise is helpful both for naps and to use all the way through the night. You can use a phone app like White Noise, or buy a dedicated white noise machine. Whatever you use, it should be played at a volume that masks both indoor and outdoor noise, but it shouldn't be so loud that it disturbs your baby's sleep.

Bedding

We all like to sleep in a comfortable bed on soft bedding. Make sure your baby's sheet is pulled tightly over the mattress and that it's not crumpled up or bunched anywhere. Your baby's cot should be sturdy and stable. Do not place your baby to sleep in a travel cot unless you are travelling.

Invest in a high-quality foam mattress covered with a waterproof mattress protector. Use 100 per cent organic cotton or bamboo cot sheets.

Sleepwear

The best type of material to dress your baby in for sleep is 100 per cent organic cotton. It's breathable, soft on baby's skin and is passed through several processes to remove germs and bacteria, helping to prevent dust mite growth.

One hundred per cent organic cotton also helps absorb moisture from your sleeping baby, keeping them dry and comfortable, helps regulate their temperature and gives them a sense of comfort.

Make sure there are no labels, which could aggravate sleep. Cut all the tags off. Also, make sure to dress your baby appropriately for the room temperature.

> **Resource for parents: the Gro Company in the UK makes some suggestions about what to dress your baby in, depending on the room temperature:**
>
> https://gro-store.com.au/blogs/news/how-to-dress-baby-for-sleep
> http://gro.co.uk/what-to-wear/

Temperature

The ideal temperature for a baby's room is between 16–20°C. Dressing your little one appropriately for their room temperature is crucial for their sleep.

When a baby's room is too warm, or they are dressed too warmly, melatonin (the sleep hormone) is inhibited, and your little one may find it much harder to fall asleep and stay asleep.

No one likes to feel stuffy and hot when they are trying to sleep, especially babies who can't move and kick the covers off or stick a leg out of bed to help themselves cool down, like we adults can. The room should not get too cold either, as that will affect sleep also.

Other sources of discomfort

If your baby is experiencing pain or discomfort somewhere in their body, they will struggle to fall or stay asleep. They might be suffering from reflux, silent reflux, eczema, allergies or food intolerances, which might be coming through from mum's diet or other foods a little one is eating.

Environmental allergies can also create skin, upper airway or digestive discomfort. Actively seek medical help to relieve their symptoms and discomfort as soon as possible, making this your main priority.

Finally, when it comes to preparing your baby's room, start early. In an ideal world, your baby's room will be ready before the baby comes.

Your baby's sleep routine

As night falls, signals of dark and quiet kick in. Babies start to settle into a concept of night and day and a twenty-four-hour rhythm. Establishing a routine (along with improving the sleep environment) will facilitate this.

Here are some ideas to improve your baby's sleep routine:

In the morning

Open the curtains on waking to allow daylight to stream through your house, helping your little one's brain and body to begin to distinguish the difference between night and day.

During the day

Engage in age-appropriate activities, get plenty of fresh air and daylight, establish a gentle structure to the day which allows both you and baby to know what comes next, such as a feed, nap or activity.

> Resource for parents: Try to spot your baby's tired signs before they become overtired:
>
> https://www.facebook.com/HappyBabyAndMe/photos/a.571281069 598295.1073741828.570781012981634/1618242978235427/?typ e=3&theater

Nap time

Naps are imperative, and it's so important to learn what your little one's tired signs are and get them to sleep when their sleep window is 'open'. It becomes much harder to put a little one down to sleep when they are overtired because their bodies begin to secrete cortisol and adrenaline (the stress hormones) to help them cope. It can also be challenging for a baby to fall asleep and stay asleep if you try and put them down to sleep too soon, as they haven't yet built up enough sleep pressure to allow them easily to drift off to sleep again.

Resource for parents: knowing your baby's awake time is key to calm, restful naps:

http://www.happybabyandme.com/why-knowing-your-babys-awake-time-is-key-to-calm-restful-naps/

Once you spot your baby's tired signs, reduce stimulation and start getting your baby ready for his nap by doing a short nap routine. Having a nap routine will help your baby understand what comes next (sleep). It also establishes positive sleep associations for the future, helps transition from 'play mode' to 'sleep mode' more easily, making it easier for your little one to calm, settle and fall asleep.

Here is Tracy's guide for 'awake times' between naps, according to the age of your baby:

Age	Awake time
0–12 weeks	45 minutes –1 hour
12–16 weeks	1 hour 15 – 1 hour 30
17–25 weeks	1 hour 30 – 2 hours
6–8 months	2 hours
9–12 months	3–4 hours
13 months–2.5 years	5–7 hours

Resource for parents: Tracy's sleep progression pyramid: http://www.happybabyandme.com/sleep-in-the-first-year-whats-normal/

Feeding

Growing babies are often hungry at least every three hours in the day. Breastfed babies often need to feed more frequently because the body digests breast milk faster than formula. Feeding your baby before sleep ensures a full tummy, which will help them settle. A good feed also helps your baby become sleepy and go to sleep more readily.

Resource for parents: Tracy's guide '39 Tips to help Your Baby Sleep Well': http://www.happybabyandme.com/free-resources/

If your baby is waking frequently and feeding to resettle, the question is why. There are so many factors that influence sleep and cause a baby to wake such as medical issues, discomfort, temperature or environment. Working out the reason for waking is paramount to both yours and baby's sleep. A rough guide for night feeds: at six months, two to three feeds; at twelve months, up to three feeds.

Preparing your baby for bedtime

Introducing a little bedtime routine helps to set the scene for sleep, show your baby what's coming next and end the day beautifully.

It should be one smooth flowing process made up of predictable steps which you repeat every single day, for example, bath, get dressed, massage, cuddle, story, lullaby and feed.

Lullaby

A lullaby acts as an excellent sleep association. By using the same lullaby every night, you help signal to your little one that it's sleep time.

Bedtime routine

Even from the very early days, a bedtime routine helps to establish positive sleep associations and will benefit both you and baby in preparing for the night ahead, but you may not see the desired results straight away. It takes up to four months for a baby's circadian rhythm (body clock) to establish and for them to fully differentiate between night and day.

Going to sleep

Babies' bodies are sensitive to light cues. Use this to your advantage in setting the scene as part of your bedtime routine.

Either after your little one's dinner or before you run the bath, do a walk around your house and set the scene, creating an ambient, calm feeling as you prepare your baby's body for sleep and bedtime.

Take it all down a notch by closing all the blinds and curtains and dimming the lights. Prepare your baby's room thoroughly, making sure it's all ready for bedtime so that when you take your little one out of the bath you have everything you need already set out, such as pyjamas, nappies, cream, sleeping bag and so on. The room should be dimly lit.

Once your baby is dressed and ready for bed, switch off all lights and feed your baby. A feed will help your baby get calm, relaxed and sleepy. It will also ensure your little one is full before going down to sleep. After your baby has fed and is sleepy, you can gently pick them up and put them down into the cot. Hopefully, at this point, baby will still be sleepy and will continue to fall asleep easily. Gently shush-pat or stroke baby's head, hair or cheek to help with falling asleep if you need to.

Babies wake for many reasons. One such reason is that baby is going through a sleep regression or about to reach a developmental milestone.

Babies go through many developmental leaps and phases that affect sleep in different ways. One is the four- or five-month sleep regression. This is the age where babies go through an incredible and massive developmental leap, and this regression is likened to that of a newborn's sleep.

Your baby may fuss a lot and seek a lot of reassurance and attention from you. With more broken nights than usual, a cranky baby who only wants to be up in your arms all day and naps that may prove tricky, it can be one of the hardest developmental leaps you'll go through in the first year.

This phase is often tiring for parents, but it is incredibly important for babies. It's really as if, during this time, they are awakening. No more the sleepy newborn baby, their senses are heightened, they can see further and are beginning to recognise faces and voices. You may find your little one less comfortable being passed around to loving friends and family and instead seeking your reassurance and comfort, making the room know it until reunited with you. Their sense of touch improves as well as their ability to move and communicate through speech (babbling) and facial expressions. It's a whole new world for them, and one that can be overstimulating and overwhelming to the senses. Once you understand this, you can more easily find understanding, compassion and empathy for your baby and see the world through his eyes, giving him all the love, reassurance and comfort he needs to get through this big leap, while he learns and makes sense of so much more.

Another phase that can often feel challenging to parents, is the eight- or nine-month separation anxiety phase. Separation anxiety peaks at around eight months. It will then come and go throughout a baby's first two years where it eases. During this time sleep is often affected, resulting in babies needing more reassurance and comfort for both night-time sleep and daytime sleep.

Night weaning

When feeding at night, keep feeds quiet and keep lighting to a minimum. It is common for a baby to have a night feed up until eighteen months, and sometimes longer depending on the child. You can attempt to gently night wean between twelve and eighteen months, but if it's a struggle, it may just mean your baby is not developmentally ready. You should wait and try a few months later.

Managing sleep when there are siblings or new babies in the house

When there are other toddlers or older children in the house, bringing a newborn into the home has additional challenges for everyone. Often the second baby (and others to follow) has to cope with more noise and excitement, and naps may happen in the pram or a sling while parents juggle the demands of the new baby and the other children. It is, without a doubt, more challenging for those with more than one little one. However, the same routine and environment tips still apply. Wearing your baby in a sling or doing naps in the buggy can be helpful when you're on the move with other children.

Go with the flow as much as possible until your youngest is a little older and sleep is more controllable.

Life is super exciting for little ones, and they need a chance to be able to transition from awake to sleep. You can't just expect them to go down for their nap or at bedtime without any pre-warning. Encouraging the right activities in the day and establishing a nap time and bedtime routine will allow your little one some time to calm and relax before sleep. Daytime sleep and night-time sleep work hand in hand. The better the daytime sleep, the better the night-time sleep.

> More advice for new mums and bubs
>
> These tips have been adapted from Tracy Newberry's blog, and she has many more gems where these came from. Visit happybabyandme. com for more tips.

Appendix B: Bedtime stories to help your kids sleep

A bedtime story before sleep can help a child feel safe, set the scene for sleep, settle daytime challenges, anxieties and bad moods and help a child build emotional literacy.

As discussed in Chapter 4, you can get creative and construct your own story for your child that will interact with their dreams, integrating resilience and coping into their thinking when they are faced with real-time problems.

You can also find books that have been written to address sleep issues or things that could be hampering good sleep routines. Here's a list of stories I recommend.

Emma Yarlett, *Orion and the Dark* (Surrey, UK: Templar, 2015).

- This story creates an opportunity to talk about bedtime fears and how to quell them.

Mylisa Larsen and Babette Cole, *How to Put Your Parents to Bed* (New York: HarperCollins, 2016).

- Once your kids practise putting you to bed, then it's your turn to put them to bed. It works like magic – be prepared to participate.

Karma Wilson and Jane Chapman, *Bear Snores On* (New York: Margaret K. McElderry Books, 2002).

- When kids watch others sleeping, being sleepy or going to sleep, it helps them feel sleepy too.

Deborah Sosin and Sara Woolley, *Charlotte and the Quiet Place* (Berkeley: Plum Blossom Books, 2015).

- Finding quiet and focusing on breathinghelps Charlotte feel better, and it will slow down your littlie too.

Mary Logue and Pamela Zagarenski, *Sleep Like a Tiger* (Boston: Houghton Mifflin Books for Children, 2012).

- This is another story that mirrors an animal slowing down and getting ready for bed.

Linda Smith and Marla Frazee, *Mrs Biddlebox* (New York: HarperCollins, 2002).

- We can all relate to being cranky and the relief once it's turned around by sleepy time. This is great story for putting daytime tensions to rest.

Margaret Wise Brown and Clement Hurd, *Goodnight Moon* (New York, NY: HarperTrophy, 2010).

- This sweet book takes bunny through the ritual of saying goodnight to everything one by one, with lovely references to the quiet, gentle sounds and the soft light – all triggers for winding down to sleep.

Sandra Boynton, *The Going to Bed Book* (New York: Little Simon, 2012).

- This book is just right for winding down the day as a joyful, silly group of animals scrub, scrub, scrub in the tub, brush, brush, brush their teeth, and finally, rock and rock and rock to sleep.

Ole Risom and Richard Scarry, *I Am a Bunny* (New York: Golden, 2010).

- A sweet, gentle story about snuggling up for winter (night-time) and waking again in spring (morning).

Lisa McCourt and Cyd Moore, *I Love You, Stinky Face* (New York: Scholastic, 2004).

- This is a vividly illustrated bedtime story that shows how the unconditional love of a mother can be tested through the relentless questions of her little boy.

Georgiana Deutsch and Ekaterina Trukhan, *10,9,8... Owls up Late!: A Countdown to Bedtime* (San Diego, CA: Silver Dolphin Books, 2017).

- One by one the little owls all fly to the nest, with lots of suggestive, sleepy words along the way and the repetitive phrase, 'It's time to rest'. It's a warm and loving story.

Chris Haughton, *Goodnight Everyone* (Somerville, MA: Candlewick Press, 2016).

- The little bear tries very hard to stay awake, but sleep becomes way too hard to resist.

Dr. Seuss, *Seuss's Sleep Book* (New York: Random House, 2012).

- The kooky drawings of billions of creatures drifting into sleep are highly suggestive, and many kids won't make it to the end of the book. This is a good one for school-aged kids.

Betsy Childs and Dan Olson, *The Girl Who Got out of Bed* (United States: Childpress Books, 2013).

- The clever dad in this story teaches the age-old counting trick to bring on the morning. Read it – as long as it does not give your little one ideas for more excuses to get out of bed!

Thank you

It takes a team to write a book.

I am indebted to my support team: my husband and sons, Andrew, Max and Sam; my son Samuel for assisting with the referencing citations; my friend Kath Martin for sage advice on referencing; my team at Well Spoken; Kerri Potter for help with developing the charts; my friends for their encouragement; Jacqui Pretty and Gina Denholm for bringing the book into reality with great support along the way; Tracy Newberry for generously sharing her experience of helping little babies sleep well; Bruno Gazzoni for graphic design.

I am grateful for the professional support from colleagues at AAMS and the AOMT, especially Marc Moeller, Samantha Weaver and Patrick McKeown; Licia Coceani Paskay for reading the manuscript and providing invaluable professional feedback as a speech language pathologist, myofunctional practitioner and dental hygienist; Dr Karen Mc Cloy AACP, Australian chapter, for help with professional editing; and my wonderful inspirational colleagues, Esther Bianchini, Joy Moeller, Ricardo Santos, Linda D'Onofrio and Diane Bahr, for endorsing my work.

Last but not least, inspiration for the book came from the phenomenal clinical work and tireless research efforts of sleep physicians worldwide, who are doing extraordinary work helping to advance the field of sleep medicine. Moreover, they happen to be some of the nicest people I have ever met. Their pleas for parents to understand more about the harm caused by sleep problems warrant translation to people's everyday lives. Thank you Dr Daniel Ng for writing the forward for *Sleep-Wrecked Kids*.

In 2014, sleep medicine pioneer Dr Christian Guilleminault connected the dots for me around airway and sleep and the critical role of myofunctional health. He lit a fire in my belly that has given me the drive to write this book. Thank you, Dr Guilleminault.

I thank you all for the part you have played in bringing this book to life.

About the author

Sharon Moore is a speech pathologist and myofunctional practitioner with four decades of clinical experience across a range of communication and swallowing disorders. She has worked in diverse clinical settings in Australia and London.

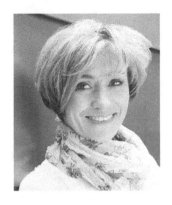

Currently, Sharon runs a private practice in Canberra for patients of all ages and is part of the transdisciplinary team for the Canberra Sleep Clinic. The integration of orofacial myofunctional principles into traditional speech pathology work allows a unique approach to managing disorders of the upper airway, including breathing, swallowing, chewing, phonation, resonance, speech, and sleep issues related to upper airway obstruction.

Sharon has a special interest in early identification of craniofacial growth anomalies in syndromic and non-syndromic children, concomitant orofacial dysfunctions and airway obstruction in sleep disorders.

Sharon believes that there has never been a more important time or medical, dental and allied health colleagues to work as a team, th the significant consequences of sleep disorders in all ages now wiuely known. Growing global medical acknowledgement of the role of myofunctional therapy in the management of sleep disorders has hailed a new era of relevance for work in the upper airway, affirming Sharon's chosen clinical direction.

She believes we have a window of opportunity to help parents get it right before kids start school.

Sharon Moore; www.sleepwreckedkids.com, FB; @the kids sleep puzzle, Instagram: sleepmattersalot. When you bought this book, something great happened in our world. We do that via our membership of the Global Giving Initiative, B1G1.com.